IV Therapy
for EMS

IV Therapy
for EMS

Randall W. Benner, M. Ed, NREMT-P
Director, Emergency Medical Technology
Youngstown State University
Youngstown, Ohio

James W. Drake, MS, NREMT-P
EMS Coordinator, Jameson Health System
New Castle, PA

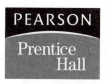

PEARSON
Prentice
Hall

Upper Saddle River, New Jersey 07458

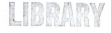
Library of Congress Cataloging-in-Publication Data
Benner, Randall W.
    IV therapy for EMS / Randall W. Benner, James W. Drake.
        p. ; cm.
    Includes index.
    ISBN 0-13-118611-6
    1. Intravenous therapy. 2. Emergency medical services. 3. Emergency medical technicians.
    [DNLM: 1. Infusions, Intravenous--methods. 2. Drug Therapy. 3.
Emergency Medical Services. WB 354 B469i 2005] I. Drake, James W. II.
Title.
    RM170.B466 2005
    615'.6--dc22

                                                                    2005007486

Publisher: Julie Levin Alexander
Publisher's Assistant: Regina Bruno
Executive Editor: Marlene McHugh Pratt
Senior Acquisitions Editor: Stephen Smith
Senior Managing Editor for Development: Lois Berlowitz
Editorial Assistant: Diane Edwards
Associate Editor: Monica Moosang
Executive Marketing Manager: Katrin Beacom
Senior Channel Marketing Manager: Rachele Strober
Marketing Coordinator: Michael Sirinides
Director of Production and Manufacturing: Bruce Johnson
Managing Editor for Production: Patrick Walsh
Production Liaison: Julie Li
Production Editor: Kelly Crooks/Techbook/GTS, York, PA Campus
Manager of Media Production: Amy Peltier
New Media Project Manager: Stephen J. Hartner
Manufacturing Manager: llene Sanford
Manufacturing Buyer: Pat Brown
Senior Design Coordinator: Christopher Weigand
Interior Designer: Mary Siener
Cover Designer: Michael Ginsberg
Cover Photo: Getty Images
Composition: Techbooks/GTS, York, PA Campus
Printing and Binding: R. R. Donnelley & Sons
Cover Printer: Phoenix Color Corporation

Photo Credits: Carl B. Leet, III / Media & Academic Computing / Youngstown State University, pp. 3, 12, 15, 27, 35, 36, 38, 40, 53, 55–59, 68–75, 77–80, 91–94, 97, 98, 115, 116, 118, 119, 129–131, 133–136, 150.

Pearson Education Ltd.
Pearson Education Singapore Pte. Ltd.
Pearson Education Canada, Ltd.
Pearson Education—Japan

Pearson Education Australia Pty. Limited
Pearson Education North Asia Ltd.
Pearson Educación de Mexico, S.A. de C.V.
Pearson Education Malaysia Pte. Ltd.

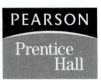
PEARSON
Prentice
Hall

10 9 8 7 6 5 4 3 2 1
ISBN 0-13-118611-6

I'd like to dedicate this work in honor of Glenn A. Benner, Jr.,
my father, my mentor, my teacher, my inspiration,
my best friend, my rock, and my greatest hero.
I miss you every day.

R. W. B.

Contents

Preface

One consistent facet of emergency medical services (EMS) is that it constantly evolves. Many skills once thought of as only imaginable have become common practice for emergency care providers across the United States. The information contained within this book is no different.

Given the climate of EMS provision in many states, it is now being recognized that the Emergency Medical Technician (EMT–Basic) can be used to initiate intravenous lines on patients and perform other common skills such as venous blood sampling. Although this book provides the EMT with the knowledge to perform this important intervention, such an intervention should occur only after there has been a structured educational component that includes knowledge testing, skill practice, and technique mastery.

Because an EMS provider cannot function without appropriate medical direction, the EMT who reads this book must also remember that the EMS system to which he or she is a part must possess appropriate medical control and treatment protocols permitting this technique. In addition, the EMS system should have a well-established quality assurance program to ensure the skills performed by the EMT are meeting both internal EMS standards and patient expectations.

Last, it is encouraged that all EMS providers, regardless of certification or licensure levels, constantly strive to better both their skills as providers and the delivery of emergency services as a whole. The weight of any EMS system rests squarely on the shoulders of those who perform these skills on a daily basis.

It is hoped by the authors that this text helps emergency care providers in continuing to achieve this purity of purpose.

Acknowledgments

The prehospital care provider now holds in his or her hands a book that is designed to provide the foundational information needed to proficiently establish intravenous lines. Although one may suspect that authoring and publishing such a text is a straightforward task, this book exists only because of the coordinated efforts of many professionals. We want to acknowledge these individuals.

First, we thank Bryan Bledsoe. Dr. Bledsoe is a person who consummates all the qualities many of us strive for in EMS. He has held, at some point, literally every position conceivable in EMS. He started as a street-level provider and progressed to become an established EMS educator and EMS program administrator. He is now a well-respected emergency physician, and is unquestionably one of the most proliferative authors for EMS and emergency medicine. He has paved the way for many and invites all to follow in his footsteps. For this and more, we are indebted to him.

Second, we are grateful to the Prentice Hall/Brady Publishing team. Like Dr. Bledsoe, they also strive for quality EMS education and have a relentless goal of providing the highest-quality EMS educational material available. Marlene Pratt, Lois Berlowitz, Monica Moosang, Julie Li, and Patrick Walsh are just as committed to the field of EMS as is any provider. How they manage all the differing tasks they have, yet maintain a clear vision of what EMS education should be, remains a mystery.

We also thank Carl Leet from Youngstown State University, who spent countless hours as the photographer for almost all the images found in this text. He is not only a professional in his trade, but also a patient man with a great sense of humor. You cannot meet him without having your spirits lifted. Kelly Crooks from TechBooks was also an invaluable contributor to this production. Her persistent efforts on this project helped bring it to fruition. Kristin Lynch, although not an author of the text, brought a great deal of improvement with her editorial expertise.

Last, but not in any measure least, we commend Gary Borman, Jack Martin, Margie Brown, Julie Brown, Theresa Farrant, and Summer Hamrick for their countless hours of remaining "perfectly still" during the photo shoots for this text. Their voluntary investment of time and expertise for this project is greatly appreciated. Also invaluable were those individuals who contributed to the text by way of manuscript review: R. Yancey Brewer, A.A.S., NREMT-P, Ridgefield, MS; E. James Cole, M.A., NREMT-P, WEMT-I, EMS-I, Lead EMS Instructor, Cleveland Clinic Health System, Cleveland, OH; Thomas L. Cook, Nursing Services Superintendent, PA Air National Guard (Retired), PA EMT Instructor, Jonesborough, TN; Michael Derme, NREMT-P, Los Angels, CA; Janice Dorey, RN, BS, EMS Education Coordinator, Advocate Christ Medical Center, Oak Lawn, IL; Jaime S. Greene, Instructor, Lake City Community College, Lake City, FL; Anthony S. Harbour, Med, NREMT-P, Virginia PHTLS State Coordinator, Richmond, VA; Robert L. Jones, REMT-P, M.A.E.D., Battalion Chief–Training, Johnson

County, Olathe, KS; David M. LaCombe, Director, National EMS Academy, Lafayette, LA; Eric T. Mayhew, A.A.S., NREMT-P, Dallas, NC; Daniel A. Palladino, A.A.S., CCEMT-P, Director of Education, Delta Ambulance, Waterville, ME; Warren Porter, BA, NREMT-P, PNCCT, EMT Coordinator, Joint Special Operations Medical Training Center, Fort Bragg, NC; Timothy J. Reitz, AS, NREMT-P, Coordinator, Conemaugh School of EMS, Johnstown, PA; Jorge Trevino, RN, Christus Santa Rosa Children's Hospital, Emergency Department Nurse Manager, San Antonio, TX; Ray Wright, Professor, EMS, Overland Park, KS. Their thoughtful and expert advice enhanced the quality of this book immeasurably.

About the Authors

Randall W. Benner, M Ed, NREMT-P

Randall Benner, instructor in the Department of Health Professions at Youngstown State University, has over 16 years of experience as an educator in emergency medical services and as a field paramedic. He serves as the Director of the Emergency Medical Technology Program at Youngstown State University and is responsible for all levels of EMS education. In addition, he actively functions as a paramedic on an advanced life support unit.

Mr. Benner has served as a contributing author for a variety of EMS textbooks, instructor resource materials, and as a medical content reviewer for EMS and allied health publications. He is also a contributing author to the revision of the U.S. Department of Transportation National Standard EMT-Intermediate and Paramedic curricula. He serves on several local, state, and national EMS committees. Mr. Benner is completing his PhD program in Curriculum and Instructional at Kent State University in Kent, Ohio.

James W. Drake, MS, NREMT-P

Jim Drake serves as the EMS Coordinator for Jameson Memorial Hospital in New Castle, Pennsylvania. Jim has been a paramedic for eleven years and involved in EMS for fifteen years. He has instructed the different levels of EMS and continues to do so at Youngstown State University, and the Community College of Allegheny County in Pittsburgh. Jim has been a contributing author for several EMS texts, and on-line continuing education programs for EMS professionals. Jim was also involved with the U.S. Department of Transportation National Standard EMT-Paramedic curricula revision.

Introduction to IV Therapy

LEARNING OBJECTIVES

By the end of this chapter, you should be able to:

- ☑ Provide a basic description of intravenous (IV) therapy and its benefit to the patient who requires emergency administration of fluids, blood, medications, or other substances
- ☑ List advantages of having the emergency medical technician (EMT) provide IV therapy in the prehospital setting
- ☑ Describe the best way to avoid clinical and legal complications associated with IV therapy

---

KEY TERMS

Advanced life support—Refers to prehospital health care providers who are capable of administering medications, cardiac monitoring, and other advanced airway and patient management skills. Paramedics are the most common ALS emergency care provider; however, in some areas, EMT–Intermediates and/or registered nurses can also provide ALS care in the prehospital setting.

ALS—See Advanced life support.

Intravenous therapy—Process by which the care provider accesses a patient's venous circulation to administer fluids or medications.

IV—See Intravenous therapy.

Medical director—The medical director is a credentialed physician who is responsible for overseeing all clinical aspects of an EMS system. The medical director directs patient care, either "online" using direct communication via radio or phone, or "offline" using written protocol or standing orders.

Case Study

You function as an EMT in a rural emergency medical services (EMS) system that permits EMTs to provide IV therapy. Within your system, there is one paramedic per shift who responds to calls in a special medic response vehicle when needed. It is midafternoon, and you are dispatched to a residence in the far reaches of the county for a 64-year-old male who is not feeling well. After a 22-minute response, you arrive at the home and find the patient lying on his side on the living room floor. As you approach, you note that the patient looks very ill and is vomiting. The initial assessment reveals him to be confused but with a patent airway and adequate breathing, albeit somewhat labored. His radial pulse is weak and slow, and his skin is cool and diaphoretic. Your partner obtains the following vital signs: pulse, 32 beats per minute; breathing, 20 breaths per minute; and blood pressure, 58/40 mm Hg. The patient lives alone and is having difficulty providing other medical information due to his confusion.

Recognizing that the patient is in severe distress, you quickly apply oxygen via a nonrebreathing face mask and call for paramedic assistance. Dispatch informs you that the paramedic has just been dispatched to another call and is unavailable. Not missing a beat, you and your partner immediately transfer the patient to the stretcher and then to the ambulance. Emergent transport is initiated to the county hospital, which is 20 minutes from your present location. Given the severity of the patient's condition and probable need for medication(s) on arrival at the hospital, you elect to start an IV. How will you proceed?

Chapter 1 presents a basic description of IV therapy, along with its role in treating the sick and the injured. The advantages of having the EMT provide IV therapy are also presented. At the end of the chapter, we return to this case and apply your knowledge.

QUESTIONS

1. What findings in the initial assessment indicate that the patient is in critical condition?
2. Even though the EMT cannot administer the emergency medications that the patient requires, why would starting an IV on the patient be beneficial?
3. Why would administering medication intravenously to this patient be better than administering the same medication orally?

■ INTRODUCTION TO IV THERAPY

IV therapy is a medical procedure in which an IV catheter is placed into a patient's vein, most commonly in the vein of the hand or arm. Accessing the patient's body by way of his or her veins is advantageous when caring for the acutely ill and injured, as well as those requiring long-term care. In

Figure 1.1. The EMT starting an IV while at a patient's house.

emergency medicine and EMS systems, IV therapy is essential in providing emergency and potentially lifesaving care to the patient in need. IV therapy allows the administration of fluids, blood, or medications directly into the circulatory system (via a vein), where they are then rapidly distributed throughout the body.

Consider the trauma patient who has lost blood that must be replaced with fluids and/or blood itself. IV access allows the fluid or blood to be directly administered where it is needed the most—the circulatory system. The same holds true for the medical patient requiring emergency medications. Administering medications through an IV quickly places them into the body and circulates them to the cells and organs where they are of benefit. There is no faster route for accessing the body or for distributing fluids and medications throughout. In the emergency situation, getting these fluids, blood, or medications into the body as quickly as possible may be the difference between a favorable and an unfavorable outcome (Figure 1.1).

Outside emergency medicine, IV therapy is a useful tool in the treatment of nonacute patients. IV access permits the repeated administration of medications, electrolytes, and nutritional substances needed to combat disease or rehabilitate an individual. Examples include those with gastrointestinal diseases who cannot receive nutritional support by mouth or individuals with cancer who require frequent infusions of medications and other agents.

On Target

IV therapy allows the administration of fluids, blood, or medications directly into the circulatory system, where they are then rapidly distributed throughout the body so as to exert their intended action.

On Target

IV therapy is the fastest and most effective way to administer and circulate fluids and medications throughout the body of a critically ill or injured patient.

Brief History of IV Therapy

IV therapy is not a new procedure, rather it has been around for some time. In the 1950s, IV therapy was only performed in a hospital by experienced physicians due to the risk for infection and the need to place a hollow metal

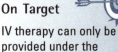

needle into a vein. However, with the advent of new IV catheters, IV therapy has gone from a procedure once reserved for the hospital to one that is routinely performed in many different settings, including the prehospital environment. Within the EMS system, IV therapy has been a standard intervention for paramedics when caring for the sick and the injured. Now, due to its proven effectiveness and the availability of EMS, some states and medical jurisdictions now permit EMTs to perform this potentially lifesaving intervention.

Advantages of EMTs Providing IV Therapy

In a system consisting exclusively of EMTs and first responders, the EMT may very well be the only prehospital care provider capable of providing IV therapy to the sick and the injured. Allowing the EMT to start and maintain IVs enables IV fluids to be delivered earlier and provides a route for lifesaving medications to be administered immediately on patient arrival to the emergency department.

In a tiered EMS system that separately responds EMTs and health care personnel capable of delivering **advanced life support** or ALS (e.g., EMT–Intermediates, paramedics, or prehospital registered nurses), allowing EMTs to start IVs holds similar benefits. IV access can be established prior to the arrival of the advanced-level care provider, therein providing the means by which the ALS provider can immediately deliver critical and potentially lifesaving care. Even in an EMS system in which the EMT and advanced-level care providers work side by side, permitting EMTs to establish IVs can allow the ALS provider to perform other critical interventions such as endotracheal intubation or the preparation of medications.

Medical Director

Like all other aspects of prehospital care provided by EMTs, IV therapy would not be possible without a medical director. A **medical director** is licensed and credentialed physician who is responsible for all clinical aspects of an EMS system, including IV therapy. The medical director decides the particular details of IV therapy, such as when an IV should be started; what materials, supplies, and solutions to use; and where on the patient's body the IV(s) should be placed. These directions can occur in the form of prewritten standing orders (offline medical direction) or require direct authorization from the medical director or other qualified physician (online medical direction). The medical director should be viewed as a resource and used accordingly. If you are having trouble with IVs, seek his or her input and consider all recommendations.

Additional Responsibilities

With the inclusion of IV therapy in the EMT's scope of practice, new responsibilities, both clinical and legal, are incurred. Although starting and maintaining IVs is relatively simple, there are associated risks and complications that the EMT must be aware of and take proactive measures to prevent or correct when identified. The EMT also has the legal responsibility to provide IV therapy in a manner that is both safe and effective, serving to benefit, not harm, the patient. To avoid clinical and legal complications, the EMT must strive to become proficient in all aspects of IV therapy. This is best accomplished through knowledge and practice.

This book presents the pertinent information required by the EMT to provide safe and effective IV therapy prior to hospitalization. Each chapter presents and discusses a different aspect of IV therapy, including the relevant anatomy and physiology, fluids used for IV therapy, site selection, equipment and supplies, and special patients for whom IV therapy presents a challenge.

Within each chapter, learning objectives, key terms, and core material related to IV therapy are presented and discussed. Additional information that enhances the EMT's knowledge and ability to provide IV therapy is presented in an Enrichment section. Review questions at the end of each chapter allow the student to test his or her knowledge.

On Target

The EMT has the legal and ethical responsibility to provide IV therapy in a manner that is both safe and effective, serving to benefit, not harm, the patient.

Case Study Follow-Up

You are managing a 64-year-old male in severe distress. Paramedic assistance is unavailable, so you have elected to transport the patient straight to the hospital. Given his slow heart rate and low blood pressure, you know that IV access is needed so critical fluids and medications can be administered. By establishing the IV en route to the hospital, the emergency department will be able to immediately administer these potentially lifesaving fluids and medications.

You quickly gather macrodrip tubing and connect it to a 1,000-milliliter bag of 0.9% normal saline solution (NSS). Looking at potential sites on the patient's hands and arms, you determine that you can get an 18-gauge IV catheter in the patient's right antecubital fossa (or AC area). You apply a venous constricting band to the right arm just above the AC area. The site is cleansed with alcohol, and the vein is punctured with the IV catheter. You see blood in the flashback chamber of the venipuncture device, and the catheter is advanced into the vein. The IV administration tubing is connected to the hub of the catheter and flow rate set. The patient's condition does not change during the remainder of the transport.

At the hospital, the patient is taken immediately to a room where fluids and medications are administered. It is rapidly determined that the patient is having a severe heart attack. He is quickly transferred to the cardiac catheterization lab for definitive care. After the catheterization, the patient spends 2 weeks in the hospital before being released to another facility for rehabilitation services.

◼ SUMMARY

EMS is a dynamic field. Consider the fact that many EMS systems allow EMTs to perform advanced airway care (endotracheal intubation, esophageal–tracheal combitube), defibrillation (automated external defibrillation), and now IV therapy. Although the prospect of placing an IV in a patient may seem intimidating, the EMT should embrace this new practice and strive to become proficient in this potentially lifesaving procedure. Doing so further expands the EMT's scope of practice and, most important, benefits the person who matters most—the patient.

REVIEW QUESTIONS

1. IV therapy can only be performed by the EMT if the medical director permits it through protocols.
   A. True
   B. False

2. IV therapy describes a medical procedure in which the tip of the IV catheter is placed into a patient's
   A. blood vessel.
   B. artery.
   C. vein.
   D. hand or arm.

3. IV therapy is a useful tool in caring for
   A. trauma patients.
   B. medical patients.
   C. patients requiring long-term care.
   D. all of the above.

4. In an EMS system where both paramedics and EMTs work side by side, one benefit of having EMTs provide IV therapy would be to
   A. free up ALS personnel for other essential tasks.
   B. provide additional tasks for the EMT to perform.
   C. decrease the need for ALS personnel such as paramedics.
   D. decrease the working relationship between EMT and ALS personnel.

5. The best way to avoid clinical and legal complications associated with IV therapy is to
   A. not start an IV unless the patient is having chest pain or shortness of breath.
   B. always allow the ALS provider to start the IV when possible.
   C. only establish an IV in patients who are not critical.
   D. gain and maintain proficiency through knowledge and practice.

Anatomy, Physiology, and Mechanism of IV Therapy

LEARNING OBJECTIVES

By the end of this chapter, you should be able to:

- ☑ Identify relevant anatomy and physiology related to IV therapy
- ☑ Describe and differentiate arteries, veins, venules, and capillaries based on anatomic and physiologic characteristics
- ☑ Explain why veins are suitable for IV therapy
- ☑ Describe the anatomy and physiology of the skin and its relationship to IV therapy
- ☑ Explain the mechanism of IV therapy and why it is an invaluable tool for care of the sick and the injured

KEY TERMS

Arteries—Large blood vessels that transport oxygen-rich blood to the capillaries and cells (blood flows away from the heart).

Arteriole—The smallest type of artery that connects larger arteries to the capillary beds. Arterioles carry oxygen-rich blood.

Capillaries—Tiny blood vessels that lie adjacent to the cells and permit the transfer of oxygen (and other important materials) to the cells.

Cardiovascular system—An organ system in the body comprised of the heart, blood, and blood vessels (arteries, veins, and capillaries).

Oxygen-poor blood—Blood that has transferred its oxygen to the cells and is returning to the right side of the heart so it can be pumped back to the lungs for reoxygenation. Oxygen-poor blood is typically carried in veins and is darker in color than oxygen-rich blood carried in arteries.

Oxygen-rich blood—Blood that has been oxygenated by the lungs and is pumped by the left side of the heart into the arteries and on to the capillaries and cells. Oxygen-rich blood is typically carried in arteries, is brighter in color than the oxygen-poor blood carried in the veins, and is under higher pressure.

Skin—Largest organ system of the body that covers the body's surface and provides numerous protective functions (also known as the integumentary system).

Valves—Structures within veins that limit the backflow of blood.

Vein—Specialized blood vessels that transport oxygen-poor blood back to the heart and lungs for reoxygenation (blood flows toward the heart).

Venule—A small vein-type vessel that connects the capillaries to veins and carries oxygen-poor blood.

Case Study

You are called to a golf course for an individual who has been stung by a bee. As you approach, you note a heavy-set 36-year-old male in moderate respiratory distress with flushed skin that is covered with hives. The scene appears safe and you have donned the appropriate body substance isolation (BSI) precautions. Your initial assessment reveals the patient to be anxious but with a patent airway and tachypneic (rapid) respirations that are slightly labored. The pulse is moderate in strength but rapid. The patient informs you that he has been stung by bees before but never suffered any sort of reaction. Quick inspection of the patient's hand shows a red and swollen area where the sting occurred. The patient tells you he plucked out the stinger prior to your arrival.

Knowing that this is a priority patient, you complete your scene size up and initial assessment as you begin administering high-flow oxygen and place the patient on the stretcher for transport to the hospital. While en route, you assemble the materials needed to start an IV and inform the patient of your intent. The patient asks you if it is really necessary because he "hates" needles and inquires as to how this will help him. Reflecting on your knowledge of the cardiovascular system and IV therapy, you prepare a response.

In Chapter 2, you learn the pertinent anatomy and physiology related to IV therapy, along with its mechanism of action within the body. At the end of the chapter, we return to this case and apply your knowledge.

QUESTIONS

1. Does the fact that the patient is heavy-set raise any concerns or challenges regarding IV therapy?
2. Given the patient's condition, would it matter if the IV were placed in an artery instead of a vein?

3. How would you respond to the patient's question asking how the IV will help him?

4. If the patient asked you whether the IV will hurt, what would you tell him?

■ INTRODUCTION

The success and proficiency with which you perform IV therapy does not just depend on technique and skill. Because IV therapy involves placing an IV catheter into a vein, you must also possess a basic understanding of the cardiovascular system (heart, blood, and blood vessels) and skin. Knowledge of the cardiovascular system, skin, and blood vessels will enable you to identify the most suitable sites for IV therapy and increase your success rate when starting an IV. Familiarity will also allow you to troubleshoot problems with the IV, while decreasing the chance for complication(s).

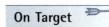

On Target

If the EMT is to become proficient with IV therapy, he or she must have a working knowledge of the relevant anatomy and physiology, as well as employ proper technique.

Cardiovascular System

IV cannulation (placement of an IV line into the body) is correctly performed when the IV catheter lies within a blood vessel called a **vein**. The term IV cannulation is literally translated into what is occurring (*intra*, within; *venous*, vein; *cannulation*, introduce cannula). Veins are part of the **cardiovascular system**, which is comprised of the heart (the pump), blood (the volume), and blood vessels (the arteries, arterioles, veins, venules, and capillaries of the body). The cardiovascular system pumps oxygen-rich blood and other essential nutrients to the cells, while transporting oxygen-poor blood to the lungs for reoxygenation and waste products to other organs (e.g., kidneys) for elimination from the body.

The process by which the cardiovascular system delivers oxygen to the cells is simple. As we breathe, oxygen enters the lungs and is transferred to **oxygen-poor blood** that has been pumped to the lungs by the right side of the heart. The now **oxygen-rich blood** is then pumped by the left side of the heart into large blood vessels called **arteries**. From the arteries, the oxygen-rich blood moves into smaller blood vessels called **arterioles**, which feed into the tiniest of blood vessels called **capillaries**. Capillaries lie next to the tissue cells and allow the transfer of oxygen from the blood to the cells (Figure 2.1). The now oxygen-poor blood then leaves the capillaries via **venules**, which increase in size and give rise to larger blood vessels called **veins**. Veins ultimately return the oxygen-poor blood to the right side of the heart, which then pumps the blood back to the lungs for reoxygenation. At this point, the entire process starts over again (Figure 2.2). If the cells of the body do not receive an adequate supply of oxygen, they will become damaged and die. Once dead, a cell cannot be revived.

Figure 2.1.
Oxygen and carbon dioxide transfer takes place at the capillary level.

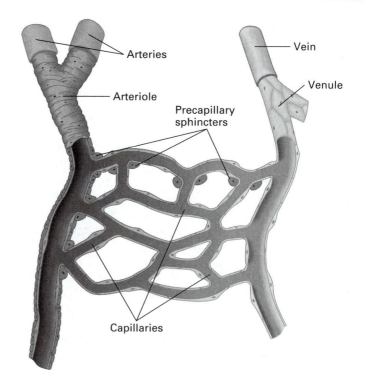

Figure 2.2. The heart and blood vessels constitute a complete, closed system.

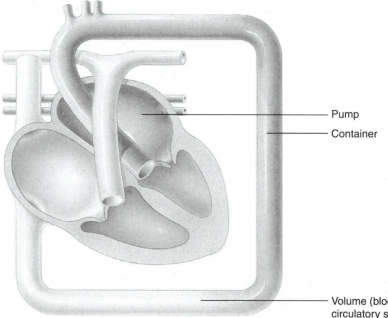

Blood Vessels

Blood vessels enable the circulation of blood throughout the body. As described previously, arteries transport oxygen-rich blood to the cells, whereas veins transport oxygen-poor blood back to the right side of the heart and lungs for reoxygenation. Because the objective of IV therapy is to place an IV catheter into a vein, it is important to understand the composition and characteristics of veins, as well as the differences between veins, venules, and arteries.

Venules are small blood vessels that connect capillaries and veins. After exiting the capillaries, oxygen-poor blood enters the venules and is moved into the veins for delivery back to the heart and lungs for reoxygenation. Compared with venules, veins are larger and more obvious on the surface of the body, particularly the extremities. It is important to note that capillaries and venules are not desirable sites for IV therapy. These vessels are too small and can be permanently damaged if the EMT attempts to place an IV here. Therefore, only veins are used for IV therapy.

The walls of veins are thin and contain less muscular tissue than arteries, making penetration with a sharp IV catheter relatively easy. Veins also contain **valves** that assist in moving blood back to the heart by limiting backflow. Knowledge of valves is important because the infusion of IV fluids into a patient may be impaired if the tip of the IV catheter somehow abuts itself at the base of the valve (Figure 2.3).

Another characteristic differentiating arteries from veins is the pressure at which the blood is transported through the respective vessels. The blood pressure in veins is much lower than the blood pressure in arteries. The lower pressure in veins allows IV fluids to flow more easily into the body by way of gravity (hanging the IV fluid bag above the patient) and makes hemorrhage easier to control if bleeding occurs when starting the IV. The blood pressure in arteries is much greater, making hemorrhage control more difficult and limiting the ease with which IV fluids can be infused into the patient.

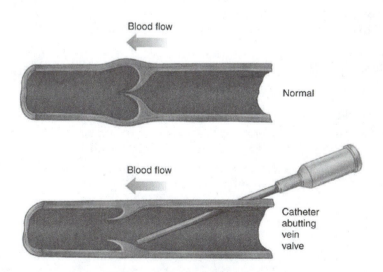

Blood flow

Normal

Blood flow

Catheter abutting vein valve

Figure 2.3. A catheter tip that is abutting a valve may fail to flow properly.

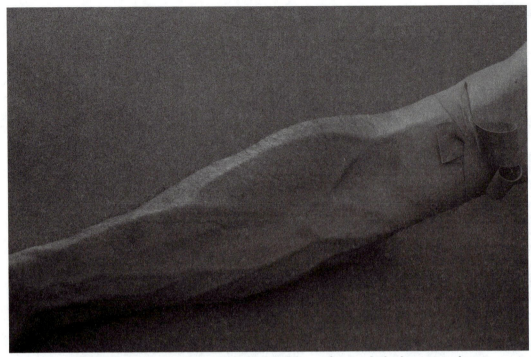

Figure 2.4. Veins lie closer to the surface of the skin, and are relatively easy to locate.

On Target

IV therapy involves placing an IV catheter in a vein, not in an artery.

Although arteries and veins lie in close proximity to each other, veins are typically found closer to the surface of the skin and arteries are found deeper. This makes veins much easier to locate and use for IV therapy (Figure 2.4). Veins and arteries also lie very close together near joints, so when starting an IV near a joint (e.g., the wrist), the EMT must exercise great caution to avoid arteries. Veins vary in size and become progressively larger the closer they get to the trunk of the body, and because the walls of the veins are thinner, they are easily distensible (can get larger). Certain techniques can be employed when starting an IV to distend the vein, making it easier to see, feel, and ultimately cannulate. (Techniques to distend veins are discussed in Chapter 6.) See Table 2.1 for a summary comparing arteries and veins.

Table 2.1. Comparing Veins and Arteries

	Vein	Artery	Significance
Walls	Thinner	Thicker	Veins are easier to penetrate with an IV catheter
Valves	Valves	No valves	Flow of IV fluids may be impaired if the end of the IV catheter is against a valve
Blood pressure	Lower	Higher	Easier to control hemorrhage in a vein if bleeding from IV therapy occurs
			Allows the IV fluids to be administered via gravity
Location in skin	Surface of skin	Deeper in skin	Veins are easier to locate and access for IV therapy

Skin

Veins most often used for prehospital IV therapy are located in the skin on the hands and arms. Because a needle must puncture the skin when initiating an IV, knowledge of the skin and its characteristics is important.

The **skin** is the largest organ of the body and consists of three layers (epidermis, dermis, and subcutaneous; Figure 2.5). The outermost layer (epidermis) provides a physical barrier between the outside world and the internal body. This layer protects us by preventing bacteria and other microorganisms from getting inside the body and causing infection. Any time the epidermis is broken, as occurs from the needle puncture necessary to start an IV, this protective function is breached, and the opportunity for microorganism invasion and infection is increased. Consequently, it is critical that you properly cleanse the skin prior to starting an IV, as well as protect the site from contamination after the IV has been established. Techniques for decontamination and protection are discussed in Chapter 6.

Most commonly, the veins used for IV therapy are in the subcutaneous layer of the skin (this layer is also referred to as subcutaneous fat). Here, the blood vessels are larger and are fairly well anchored by the subcutaneous tissue. To reach these vessels with the IV catheter, however, you must first puncture through the epidermal and dermal layers of the skin. Although the epidermis is comprised primarily of compacted, dead skin cells, the dermis contains numerous sensory fibers that allow us to perceive sensations such as hot, cold, pressure, and pain (Figure 2.6). Because IV therapy involves inserting a sharp catheter through the skin, the patient *will feel pain*. Careless technique when starting an IV not only causes undue pain, but can also permanently damage nerve endings and blood vessels within these layers of the skin.

The amount of subcutaneous fat that the skin contains depends on the individual person and area of the body. In regions such as the dorsum

On Target

Because the dermal layer of the skin contains pain receptors, the patient will experience temporary pain as the IV catheter is inserted through the skin and into the vein.

Figure 2.5. Layers of the skin.

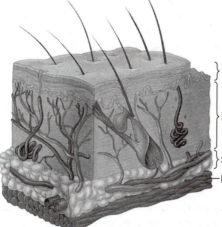

} Epidermis

} Dermis

} Subcutaneous fatty tissue

— Muscle fibers

Figure 2.6.
Structures within the layers of the skin.

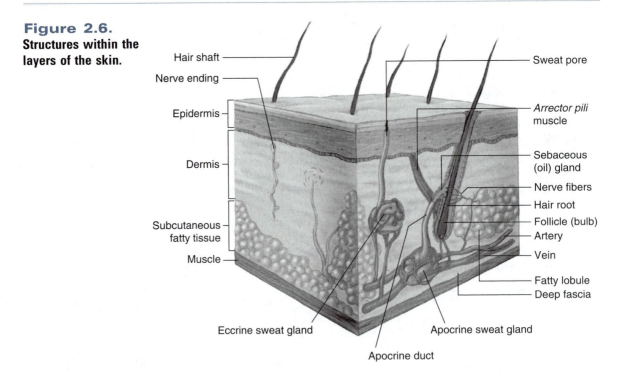

- Hair shaft
- Nerve ending
- Epidermis
- Dermis
- Subcutaneous fatty tissue
- Muscle
- Sweat pore
- Arrector pili muscle
- Sebaceous (oil) gland
- Nerve fibers
- Hair root
- Follicle (bulb)
- Artery
- Vein
- Fatty lobule
- Deep fascia
- Eccrine sweat gland
- Apocrine sweat gland
- Apocrine duct

On Target

As the amount of subcutaneous fat increases, veins typically become more difficult to locate.

(back or posterior surface) of the hand, forearm, and ventral (front or anterior) surface of the antecubital region, the amount of subcutaneous tissue tends to be less, making veins more apparent and easier to access. As the amount of subcutaneous tissue increases, veins can become "buried" and more difficult to locate (Figures 2.7a and 2.7b).

Mechanism of IV Therapy

IV therapy provides direct access into the body via the cardiovascular system (specifically, by way of the veins). As such, IV therapy is the most effective means to get fluids and medications to the exact place they are required—the cells and organs. If a person is severely dehydrated or has lost blood, IV therapy allows fluid or blood to be quickly replaced by direct administration back into the circulatory system. IV administration of medications enables them to quickly get to the exact cells and organs where they are of benefit. (Even though the EMT will probably not be administering medications, he or she may be the one initiating the IV for use by paramedics or hospital personnel.) Furthermore, once an IV is established, it can be used over the course of 24 to 72 hours (in most hospitals) for the repeated administration of fluids, blood, electrolytes, medications, and even nutritional supplements.

On Target

Because IV therapy provides direct access to the cardiovascular system through a vein, it is the most rapid means by which a fluid or medication can be administered and circulated throughout the body.

Consequently, this makes IV therapy an effective and lifesaving intervention when caring for the sick or injured patient.

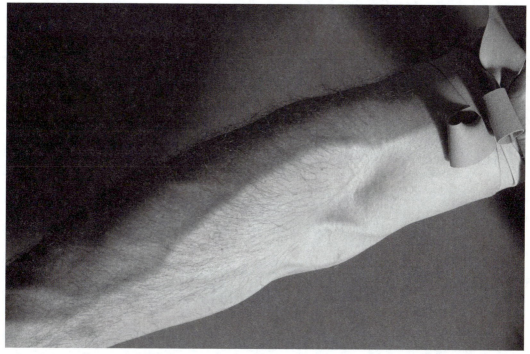

Figure 2.7a. Tangential lighting may help identify veins that are otherwise difficult to find.

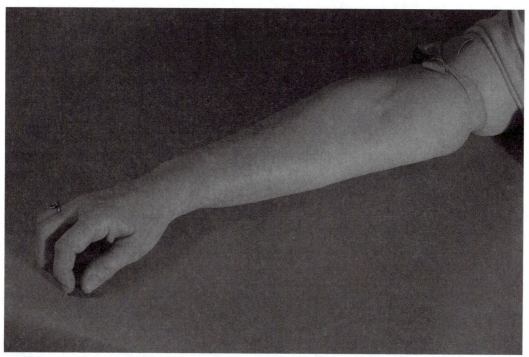

Figure 2.7b. Increased adipose deposition in the tissues can effectively hide veins needed for IV therapy.

Enrichment

Veins can be classified as either peripheral or central (Figure 2.8). Peripheral veins are located close to the surface of the body, most often on the hands, arms, legs, and neck. Because they are readily accessible, peripheral veins are used for prehospital IV therapy.

Central veins are located deep within the body. These veins are large and can also be used for IV therapy. IVs placed in central veins are called "central lines" and can be left in place much longer than an IV in a peripheral

Figure 2.8. Common locations for venous access—both central and peripheral locations.

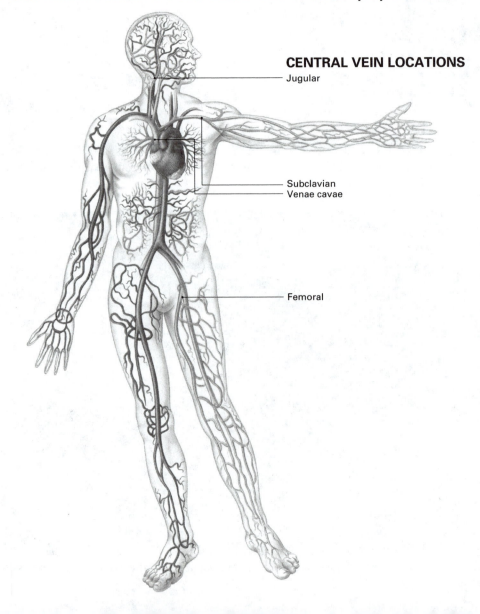

CENTRAL VEIN LOCATIONS

Jugular

Subclavian
Venae cavae

Femoral

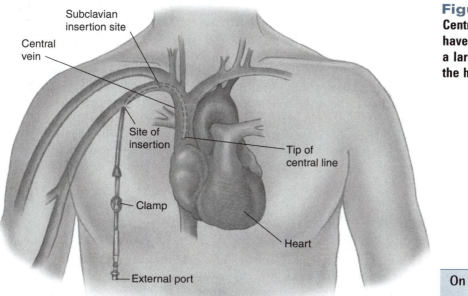

Figure 2.9.
Central venous lines have the tip resting in a large vein, close to the heart.

vein. Patients with chronic diseases or other conditions requiring long-term IV therapy often have a central line placed while they are in the hospital (Figure 2.9). Due to the higher risks and complexity associated with placement, central IVs are only established in the hospital setting by experienced physicians. Although the EMT will never start a central IV line, you may encounter a sick or injured patient with one in place.

On Target

Because IVs placed in central veins can be left in place much longer than IVs placed in peripheral veins, they are often found in patients who have chronic illnesses requiring long-term treatment.

Case Study Follow–Up

You are transporting a 36-year-old male suffering from an allergic reaction to a bee sting. In the process of assembling the materials needed for IV therapy, the patient asks you why an IV is necessary and how it will benefit him. Reflecting on your knowledge of the cardiovascular system and blood vessels, you inform him that he is having an allergic reaction and will most likely require medications to counter the effects of the bee sting. These medications can be administered through the IV and quickly transported by his blood to the exact areas of the body where they are needed. You continue to inform him that the IV route is the fastest and most effective way to administer these medications.

When starting the IV, you take care to look for a suitable vein and avoid any arteries that may lie nearby. Because the patient is heavy-set, you realize that his veins will most likely be harder to locate due to increased amounts of subcutaneous tissue. After finding a suitable vein, you inform the patient that you are cleansing the skin to reduce the risk of infection. You state that he will feel a little pain as the needle is inserted through the skin and into the vein. The IV is established, but the infusion of fluid into the patient is slow. Realizing that the tip of the IV catheter may be against a valve or the wall of the blood vessel (if the vein has a sharp turn to it), you gently pull the catheter back and observe an increase in the flow of IV fluid.

At the hospital, the emergency department nurses administer Benadryl and a steroid through the IV you established. Within half an hour, about the time you take to complete your prehospital care report (PCR) and prepare the ambulance for the next call, you learn the patient's condition has improved and he will eventually be released. One week later, the patient stops by the station and informs your supervisor that you "really know your stuff" and extends his personal thanks for your help.

■ SUMMARY

Knowledge of the cardiovascular system, as well as the differences between arteries, veins, capillaries, and venules, is an important aspect of IV therapy, as is an appreciation of the skin's characteristics and functions. Understanding this anatomy and physiology increases the chance of successfully placing an IV, while decreasing the opportunity for complications (e.g., accidental puncture of an artery or infection caused by failure to cleanse the skin prior to initiation). This information is also critical to understanding the mechanism of IV therapy and enables the EMT to better appreciate the indications and uses of this intervention. Ultimately, knowledge in this area will enhance professionalism and patient care.

REVIEW QUESTIONS

1. An IV is properly established when the IV catheter is placed in a/an _____.
   A. artery
   B. venule
   C. capillary
   D. vein

2. _____ are more suitable than _____ for IV therapy because they lie near the surface of the skin and have less muscular tissue.
   A. Veins, arteries
   B. Arteries, veins
   C. Capillaries, veins
   D. Venules, veins

3. In veins, what function does a valve serve?
   A. Prevents blood from flowing to the right side of the heart
   B. Limits the backflow of blood
   C. Obstructs blood from leaving the cardiovascular system
   D. Valves do not serve any beneficial function in veins

4. When starting an IV, it is advantageous to place the IV catheter near a valve to increase the flow of IV fluid into the patient.
   A. True
   B. False

5. What type of blood vessel is large and has thick muscular walls that facilitate the transport of oxygen-rich blood under high pressure?
   A. Capillary
   B. Artery
   C. Venule
   D. Vein

6. In regions such as the hands and lower forearms, the amount of subcutaneous fat tends to be less, making veins more apparent and easier to locate.
   A. True
   B. False

7. Why is IV therapy an effective means to get fluids, medications, and other solutions into and throughout the body?
   A. Direct access into the arteries will get the fluids, medications, and other solutions to the heart much faster
   B. Placement of fluids, medications, and other solutions into the cardiovascular system bypasses the cells and organs
   C. Fluids, medications, and other solutions are absorbed through the skin prior to entering the cardiovascular system
   D. Delivery of fluids, medications, and other solutions into the cardiovascular system provides a direct route to the cells and organs

8. Why would the patient feel pain when starting an IV?
   A. Pain receptors in the capillaries
   B. Nerve receptors in the dermal layer of the skin
   C. Pain receptors in the epidermis
   D. Damage to a valve located within an artery

9. Peripheral veins are good for IV access because they are located in the epidermal layer of the skin.
   A. True
   B. False

10. In what location of the body do arteries and veins lie closer together, possibly resulting in accidental arterial puncture if precautions are not taken?
    A. Forearm
    B. Neck
    C. Hand
    D. Joints

Intravenous Fluid Selection

LEARNING OBJECTIVES

By the end of this chapter, you should be able to:

- ☑ Describe and differentiate colloid and crystalloid IV fluids
- ☑ Understand osmosis as it pertains to water movement with IV therapy
- ☑ Define tonicity and the actions of isotonic, hypotonic, and hypertonic crystalloids in the body
- ☑ Identify the three most common IV solutions used in the prehospital setting, and classify them as isotonic, hypotonic, or hypertonic
- ☑ Describe how an IV fluid is packaged and important information located on the label of the IV fluid

KEY TERMS

5% Dextrose in water—A carbohydrate solution that uses glucose (sugar) as the solute dissolved in sterile water. Five percent dextrose in water is packed as an isotonic solution but becomes hypotonic once in the body because the glucose (solute) dissolved in sterile water is metabolized rapidly by the body's cells.

Colloid solutions—IV fluids containing large proteins and molecules that tend to stay within the vascular space (blood vessels).

Crystalloid solutions—IV fluids containing varying concentrations of electrolytes.

D_5W—See 5% dextrose in water.

Extracellular space—Space outside the cells consisting of the intravascular and interstitial spaces.

Hypertonic crystalloid—A crystalloid solution that has a higher concentration of electrolytes than the body plasma.

Hypotonic crystalloid—A crystalloid solution that has a lower concentration of electrolytes than the body plasma.

Intracellular space—Space within the cells.

Intravascular volume—Volume of blood contained within the blood vessels.

Intravenous fluids—Chemically prepared solutions that are administered to a patient through the IV site.

Isotonic crystalloid—A crystalloid solution that has the same concentration of electrolytes as the body plasma.

Lactated Ringer's—An isotonic crystalloid solution containing the solutes sodium chloride, potassium chloride, calcium chloride, and sodium lactate, dissolved in sterile water (solvent).

LR—See Lactated Ringer's.

Normal saline solution—An isotonic crystalloid solution that contains sodium chloride (salt) as the solute, dissolved in sterile water (solvent). The specific concentration for normal saline solution is 0.9%.

NS—See Normal saline solution.

NSS—See Normal saline solution.

Osmosis—The movement of water across a semipermeable membrane from an area of lower solute concentration to an area of higher solute concentration. This movement of water allows the equalization of the solute-to-solution ratio across the membrane.

Oxygen-carrying solutions—Chemically prepared solutions that can carry oxygen to the cells.

Plasma—Fluid surrounding the cells of the body.

Ringer's lactate—See Lactated Ringer's.

Solute—Particles that are dissolved in the sterile water (solvent) of an IV fluid.

Solvent—The liquid portion of an IV solution into which a solute is dissolved. The most common solvent is sterile water.

Total body water—Water contained within the cells, around the cells, and in the bloodstream. Water makes up about 60% of the body's weight.

Case Study

You are staffing a first aid center for the city's 5-kilometer run for charity. With the temperature at 96°F and the humidity at 92%, the first aid center is overwhelmed with patients suffering from dehydration. Because IV therapy is within your scope of practice, the lead physician instructs you to start an IV and administer IV fluid to a 32-year-old female who is seriously dehydrated and extremely weak.

After accessing the patient's airway, breathing, and circulation and applying high-flow oxygen, you proceed to the medical supply area to get the IV fluid. There you find a variety of fluids, including isotonic crystalloids, hypertonic crystalloids, hypotonic crystalloids, and a refrigerator of colloid solutions. What fluid will you select for this patient?

In this chapter, different types of IV fluids are presented, along with their specific actions within the body. The manner in which IV fluids are packaged is also discussed. At the end of the chapter, we return to this case and apply our knowledge.

QUESTIONS

1. How might the clinical condition of dehydration affect your ability to locate and access a vein for IV therapy?
2. Would 5% dextrose in water (D_5W) be an acceptable IV fluid to use for the rehydration of this patient?
3. If 0.9% NSS was not available, what other isotonic crystalloid would be acceptable to use in its place?

■ INTRODUCTION

Intravenous fluids are chemically prepared solutions that are administered to the patient. They are tailored to the body's needs and used to replace lost fluid and/or aid in the delivery of IV medications. For patients that do not require immediate fluid or drug therapy, the continuous delivery of a small amount of IV fluid can be used to keep a vein patent (open) for future use. IV fluids come in different forms and have different impacts on the body. Therefore, it is important to have an understanding of the different types of IV fluids, along with their indications for use.

How Intravenous Fluids Are Created

On Target

Not all IV fluids are the same. Different IV fluids have different actions within the body.

There are several types of IV fluids that have different effects on the body. Some IV fluids are designed to stay in the intravascular space (*intra*, within; *vascular*, blood vessels) to increase the **intravascular volume,** or volume of circulating blood. Other IV fluids are specifically designed so the fluid leaves the intravascular space and enters the interstitial and intracellular spaces. Still others are created to distribute evenly between the intravascular, interstitial, and cellular spaces. The properties that an IV solution has within the body depends on how it is created and the specific materials it contains. It also determines the best type of IV solution to use in relation to the patient's needs.

The majority of an IV solution is sterile water. Chemically, water is referred to as a "solvent." A solvent is a substance that dissolves other materials called "solutes." Within IV solutions, the solutes can be molecules called electrolytes (charged particles such as sodium, potassium, and chloride) and/or other larger compounds such as proteins or molecules.

Together, the **solvent** (water) and **solutes** (electrolytes, proteins, or other molecules dissolved in the water) create the IV solution. Consider a cup of coffee to which sugar is added for sweetness. The coffee is the solvent, which dissolves the solute sugar.

On Target

IV fluids are comprised of solutes dissolved in a solvent.

Intravenous Fluids

IV fluids come in four different forms:

- Colloid solutions
- Crystalloid solutions
- Blood and blood products
- Oxygen-carrying solutions

Understanding these IV fluids is important because each has a different impact on the body and particular indications for use:

- **Colloid Solutions. Colloid solutions** are IV fluids that contain solutes in the form of large proteins or other similarly sized molecules. The proteins and molecules are so large that they cannot pass through the walls of the capillaries and onto the cells. Accordingly, colloids remain in the blood vessels for long periods of time and can significantly increase the intravascular volume (volume of blood). The proteins also have the ability to attract water from the cells into the blood vessels. However, although the movement of water from the cells into the bloodstream may be beneficial in the short term, continual movement in this direction can cause the cells to lose too much water and become dehydrated.

  Colloids are useful in maintaining blood volume, but their use in the field is limited. Colloids are expensive, have specific storage requirements, and have a short shelf life. This makes their use more suitable in the hospital setting. However, familiarity is important because in a mass casualty incident the EMT may be required to assist with the administration of colloids either in a field hospital or during the transport of critically injured patients. Commonly used colloid solutions include plasma protein fraction, salt-poor albumin, dextran, and hetastarch. To learn more about colloidal solutions, the EMT should consult a critical care or paramedic textbook.

On Target

Although colloids are an effective IV solution for increasing a patient's blood volume, their expense and specific storage requirements limit their use in the prehospital setting.

- **Crystalloid Solutions. Crystalloid solutions** are the primary fluid used for prehospital IV therapy. Crystalloids contain electrolytes (e.g., sodium, potassium, calcium, chloride) but lack the large proteins and molecules found in colloids. Crystalloids come in many preparations and are classified according to their "tonicity."

  A crystalloid's tonicity describes the concentration of electrolytes (solutes) dissolved in the water, as compared with that of body **plasma** (fluid surrounding the cells). When the crystalloid contains the same amount of electrolytes as the plasma, it has the same concentration and is referred to as "isotonic" (*iso,* same; *tonic,* concentration). If a crystalloid contains more electrolytes than the body plasma, it is more concentrated and referred to as "hypertonic" (*hyper,* high; *tonic,* concentration).

Figure 3.1.
Locations of intra-cellular, interstitial, and intravascular spaces in a capillary bed.

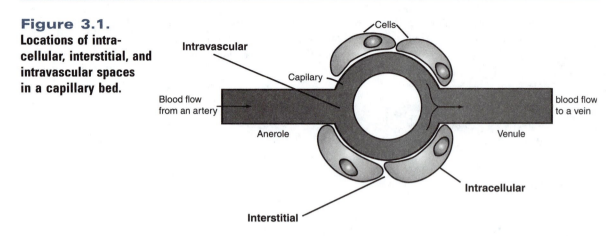

Consider the example of coffee and sugar. The more sugar that is added to the coffee, the more concentrated the sugar becomes relative to the amount of coffee, and the sweeter tasting the coffee becomes.

Conversely, when a crystalloid contains fewer electrolytes than the plasma, it is less concentrated and referred to as "hypotonic" (*hypo,* low; *tonic,* concentration). The less sugar a cup of coffee contains, the lower its concentration or tonicity, and the less sweet the coffee may taste.

Depending on their concentration, crystalloids can affect the distribution of water within the body. To better understand this, the EMT must be familiar with what **total body water** (TBW) is. TBW describes the entire amount of water contained within the body and accounts for approximately 60% of body weight. It is distributed among the intracellular and extracellular compartments. The **intracellular space** is the space within all the body cells (*intra,* within; *cellular,* cell). The **extracellular space** is the space outside the cells (*extra,* outside; *cellular,* cells). The extracellular compartment can be further divided into the intravascular space (space within the blood vessels) and the interstitial space (space between the cells but not within the blood vessels) (Figure 3.1).

The different compartments are separated by membranes through which the body water can easily pass. As a general rule, body water is pulled toward the solution with a higher concentration of dissolved molecules. The movement of water across a semipermeable membrane that selectively allows certain particles to pass while inhibiting others (i.e., a capillary wall or cellular wall) is known as **osmosis.** The osmotic movement of water occurs as the body attempts to create a balance between the different solute concentrations that exist on either side of a semipermeable membrane. What this means is that the water will easily cross the semipermeable membrane from the side that has a lower concentration of particles to the side that has a higher concentration of particles. The net movement of water stops when each side of the membrane becomes equal in its concentration of particles. With this in mind, isotonic, hypertonic, and hypotonic IV fluids cause the following shifts of body water:

- **Isotonic.** **Isotonic crystalloids** have a tonicity *equal* to the body plasma. When administered to a normally hydrated patient, isotonic

On Target

Through osmosis, water is pulled from an area of lower solute concentration to an area of higher solute concentration.

On Target

Isotonic crystalloids have a tonicity that is equal to the plasma in the body. When administering an isotonic crystalloid, the fluid will distribute evenly between the intravascular space and cells.

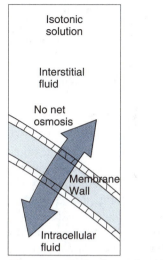

Figure 3.2. Isotonic solutions do not result in any significant fluid shifts across cellular or vascular membranes.

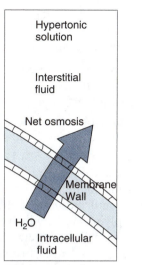

Figure 3.3. A hypertonic solution given IV will draw fluids from the cells and interstitial spaces into the vasculature.

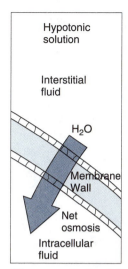

Figure 3.4. A hypotonic solution given IV will cause fluids to leave the vasculature for the interstitial and intracellular spaces.

crystalloids do not cause a significant shift of water between the blood vessels and the cells. Thus, there is no (or minimal) osmosis occurring (Figure 3.2).

- **Hypertonic.** **Hypertonic crystalloids** have a tonicity *higher* than the body plasma. The administration of a hypertonic crystalloid causes water to shift from the extravascular spaces into the bloodstream, increasing the intravascular volume. This osmotic shift occurs as the body attempts to dilute the higher concentration of electrolytes contained within the IV fluid by moving water into the intravascular space (Figure 3.3).

- **Hypotonic.** **Hypotonic** crystalloids have a tonicity *lower* than the body plasma. The administration of a hypotonic crystalloid causes water to shift from the intravascular space to the extravascular space, and eventually into the tissue cells. Because the IV solution being administered is hypotonic, it creates an environment where the extravascular spaces have higher concentrations of electrolytes. The osmotic change results in the body moving water from the intravascular space to the cells in an attempt to dilute the electrolytes (Figure 3.4).

Of the different types of IV solutions, crystalloids are the mainstay of IV therapy in the prehospital setting. The particular type of IV crystalloid selected depends on the patient's needs, based on the osmotic movement of water as described previously, a person with a low volume of blood may benefit from a hypertonic or isotonic crystalloid solution that will increase blood volume, whereas a hypotonic crystalloid would be more appropriate for a person suffering from cellular

On Target

Hypertonic crystalloids have a tonicity that is greater than the plasma in the body. When administering a hypertonic crystalloid, the fluid will pull water from the cells into the intravascular space (blood vessels).

On Target

Hypotonic crystalloids have a tonicity that is less than the plasma in the body. When administering a hypotonic crystalloid, the fluid will quickly move from the intravascular space (blood vessels) into the cells.

dehydration. The EMS system's medical director will determine which crystalloids will be used for prehospital IV therapy.

The most common isotonic solutions used in prehospital care are:

- **Lactated Ringer's.** Lactated Ringer's (LR) is an isotonic crystalloid that contains sodium chloride, potassium chloride, calcium chloride, and sodium lactate in sterile water.

- **Normal saline solution.** Normal saline solution (NSS) is an isotonic crystalloid that contains 0.9% sodium chloride (salt) in sterile water.

- **5% Dextrose in water.** 5% Dextrose in water (D_5W) is packaged as an isotonic carbohydrate (sugar solution) that contains glucose (sugar) as the solute. D_5W is useful in keeping a vein open by delivering a small amount of the fluid over a long period of time and/or supplying sugar, which is used by the cells to create energy. However, once D_5W enters the body, the cells rapidly consume the glucose. This leaves primarily water and causes IV fluid to become hypotonic in relation to the plasma surrounding the cells. Accordingly, the now hypotonic solution causes an osmotic shift of water to and from the bloodstream and into the cells.

On Target

The isotonic fluids 0.9% NSS and LR are the most common IV fluids used in the prehospital setting.

In the prehospital setting, LR and NSS are commonly used for fluid replacement because of their immediate ability to expand the volume of circulating blood. However, over the course of about 1 hour, approximately two-thirds of these IV fluids eventually leave the blood vessels and move into the cells. Some authorities recommend that for every 1 liter of blood lost, 3 liters of an isotonic crystalloid be administered for replacement. This is only a guide, and the volume of IV fluid administered should be based on medical direction or local protocol, as well as the patient's clinical needs and response to fluid administration.

- **Blood and Blood Products.** Blood and blood products (e.g., platelets, packed red blood cells, plasma) are the most desirable fluids for replacement. Unlike colloids and crystalloids, the hemoglobin (in the red blood cells) carries oxygen to the cells. Not only is the intravascular volume increased, but the fluid administered can also transport oxygen to the cells. Blood, however, is a precious commodity and must be conserved to benefit people most in need. Its use in the field is generally limited to aeromedical services or mass casualty incidents. The universal compatibility of O-negative blood makes it the ideal choice for administration in emergent situations. To learn more about blood and blood products, consult a critical care or paramedic textbook.

- **Oxygen-Carrying Solutions.** Oxygen-carrying solutions are synthetic fluids that carry and deliver oxygen to the cells. These fluids, which remain experimental, show promise for the prehospital care of patients who have experienced severe blood loss or are otherwise suffering from hypovolemia. It is hoped that oxygen-carrying solutions will be similar to crystalloid solutions in cost, storage capability, and ease of administration, and be capable of carrying oxygen, which presently only accomplished with blood or blood products.

Intravenous Fluid Packaging

Most IV fluids are packaged in soft plastic or vinyl bags of various sizes (10, 50, 100, 250, 500, 1,000, 2,000, and 3,000 milliliters) (Figure 3.5). The EMT will most likely be using 250-, 500-, and 1,000-milliliter bags. Some IV solutions are premixed with medications that are not compatible with plastic or vinyl and must be packaged in glass bottles. Glass bottles are not common to prehospital IV therapy but may be encountered during interfacility or critical care transports.

Every IV fluid container contains a label. The label provides important information relating to the IV solution including:

- Type of IV fluid (by name and by type of solutes contained within).
- Amount of IV fluid (expressed in milliliters or "ml").
- Expiration date.

Carefully read the label to ensure you are administering the correct IV solution. Many different IV fluids are packaged in similar containers, including those containing premixed medications. Administering an inappropriate IV fluid may be detrimental or even fatal to the patient, resulting in disciplinary and/or legal action. Like any other medication, IV solutions have a shelf life and must not be used after their expiration date (Figure 3.6).

The IV fluid container contains a medication injection site and administration set port. Both ports are located on the bottom of the IV bag when

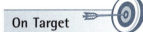

On Target

To ensure the right patient receives the right IV fluid, it is imperative that the EMT read the label of the IV container prior to preparing and administering the fluid!

Figure 3.5. Different volumes of IV bags are used in the prehospital evironment.

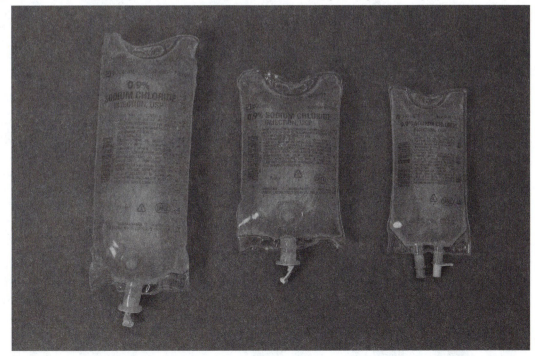

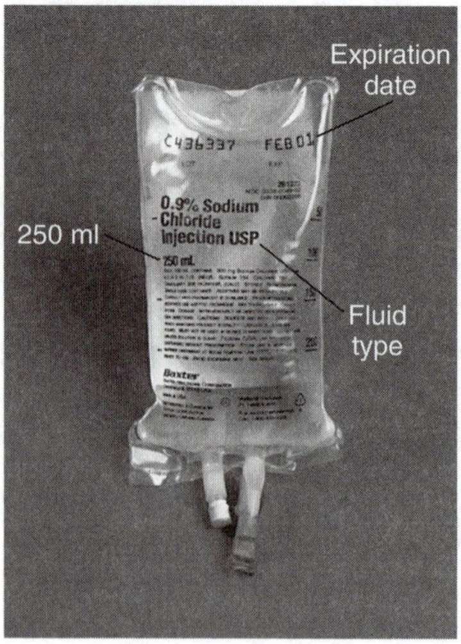

Figure 3.6. The EMT must be able to recognize the various labels and information printed on the IV bag.

holding it upright. The medication injection port permits the injection of medication into the fluid for use by advanced life support (ALS) or hospital personnel after the EMT has initiated the IV. The administration set port receives the spike from the IV administration set (IV tubing) (see Figure 3.6). Different types of IV administration sets are discussed in Chapter 5.

Case Study Follow-Up

You have been asked to start an IV and administer IV fluid to a 32-year-old female who is dehydrated after running a marathon in hot and humid weather. In the medical supply area, you find a variety of IV fluids, including isotonic crystalloids, hypertonic crystalloids, hypotonic crystalloids, and a refrigerator of colloid solutions.

Knowing that the patient requires IV fluid to both increase the blood volume and rehydrate the cells, you look at the shelf containing isotonic crystalloids. On the shelf, you find and retrieve a 1,000-milliliter bag of 0.9% NSS. Your assistant, who is not an EMT, asks why you did not use any of the other solutions. You inform him that a colloid solution and a hypertonic crystalloid would just increase the blood volume by pulling water into the blood vessels from the cells. Although the blood volume would be increased, the cells could become further dehydrated. You continue by stating that the low concentration of solutes in a hypotonic solution would cause water to shift from within the blood vessels to the cells. This would be advantageous to the cells, but the volume of blood would not be increased and may even be further reduced.

After administering the IV fluid to the patient, she states that she feels much better and is eventually released by the physician. Later, your assistant tells you that he is so impressed with your knowledge that he has decided to enroll in the next EMT class.

■ SUMMARY

There are several different types of fluids used for IV therapy. Depending on their specific type and makeup, IV fluids can cause the shift and redistribution of body water between the intracellular and extracellular compartments. Therefore, it is important that the EMT has a basic understanding of the different IV fluids and choose the fluid most appropriate to the patient's needs. Because most IV fluids are packaged in similar-looking plastic bags, it is imperative that the EMT to carefully read the label on the bag to ensure the right fluid has been selected. Administering an inappropriate IV fluid can result in undesirable complications, as well as less than optimal patient care.

REVIEW QUESTIONS

1. All IV fluids have the same impact within the body.
   A. True
   B. False

2. In an IV solution, the sterile water into which electrolytes, proteins, or other materials are dissolved is referred to as the
   A. tonicity.
   B. solvent.
   C. solute.
   D. concentration.

3. Which of the following are types of IV solutions?
   A. Colloids
   B. Crystalloids
   C. Blood
   D. All of the above are types of IV solutions

4. An IV solution contains the electrolyte sodium. Which of the following statements is true concerning the sodium?
   A. The sodium is the solution.
   B. The sodium is the solute.
   C. The sodium is the solvent.
   D. All of the above are true concerning the sodium.

5. You are administering an IV solution that contains large proteins and molecules. As such, what category of IV solution are you administering?
   A. Extravascular solution
   B. Crystalloid solution
   C. Colloid solution
   D. Hypotonic crystalloid solution

6. The most commonly administered IV fluid given prehospitally is a colloid solution.
   A. True
   B. False

7. A crystalloid solution typically contains sterile water and
   _____.
   A. proteins
   B. blood
   C. oxygen crystals
   D. electrolytes

8. Which of the following best describes a hypertonic solution?
   A. Concentration higher than the body plasma
   B. Concentration lower than the body plasma
   C. Contains less electrolytes than the body plasma
   D. Contains more oxygen crystals than the body plasma

9. Match the following IV solutions to their description:
   ____ Hypertonic crystalloid   A. Concentration the same as the body plasma

   ____ Isotonic crystalloid   B. Concentration less than the body plasma

   ____ Hypotonic crystalloid   C. Concentration greater than the body plasma

10. Identify the crystalloid solution.
    A. Hetastarch
    B. Lactated Ringer's
    C. Blood
    D. Oxygen-carrying solution

11. The most commonly used fluids for prehospital IV therapy are
    A. colloids, crystalloids, and blood
    B. lactated Ringer's, blood, and 5% dextrose in water (D_5W)
    C. blood, 5% dextrose in water (D_5W), and sterile water
    D. Normal saline solution and lactated Ringer's

12. It is important to read the label on every IV bag because
    A. different IV solutions are packaged similarly.
    B. the label contains the expiration date of the IV fluid.
    C. the name of the IV solution is on the label.
    D. all of the above are reasons why the EMT should read the label on every IV bag.

13. The tonicity of an IV solution is described as
    A. the amount of oxygen that it can carry to the cells.
    B. the type of water contained within the solution.
    C. the concentration of the solution as compared with the body plasma.
    D. the amount of blood contained within the solution.

14. As long as an isotonic solution is used, it makes no significant difference if the solution contains glucose molecules instead of electrolytes.
    A. True
    B. False

15. Osmosis is the movement of water from an area of high concentration of molecules and/or electrolytes to an area containing a lower concentration of molecules and/or electrolytes.
    A. True
    B. False

Intravenous Site Selection

LEARNING OBJECTIVES

By the end of this chapter, you should be able to:

- ☑ List the most common sites used for prehospital IV access
- ☑ Describe the importance of selecting an appropriate site and vein for IV therapy
- ☑ List factors used to determine what site(s) is most suitable for IV access
- ☑ Describe the importance of using techniques that facilitate vein engorgement when preparing to place an IV
- ☑ Identify conditions that contraindicate or preclude the EMT from starting an IV in the immediate area or particular extremity

KEY TERMS

AC—See Antecubital fossa.

Antecubital fossa—Area containing large veins located at the anterior surface of the elbow.

Bifurcated vein—A larger common vein formed when two smaller veins join together.

Dialysis shunt—Surgically placed device that joins an artery directly with a vein (commonly in the arm) and allows a patient with renal failure to be attached to a dialysis machine.

Edema—Fluid collection in the interstitial spaces between the cells (also referred to as swelling).

EJ—See External jugular vein.

External jugular vein—Large vein located on the lateral surface of either side of the neck.

Mastectomy—Surgical removal of a breast.

Case Study

You and your partner have been called to the home of a 62-year-old female complaining of generalized weakness and nausea. The scene is safe, and the patient is found seated in a chair in the living room. Your assessment reveals no immediate life threats to the airway, breathing, or circulation, and her vital signs are pulse, 72 beats per minute; respirations, 16 per minute; and blood pressure, 134/80 mm Hg. However, because the patient has a history of diabetes and has had a previous heart attack, you realize that she has several risk factors that predispose her to rapid deterioration. The patient also states that she has a medical history of breast cancer and hypertension, which is controlled by medications. Dispatch informs you that an ambulance with paramedics has been dispatched and will meet you en route to the hospital.

The physical assessment and vital signs indicate the patient is currently stable, and after placing the patient on oxygen, you move her onto the stretcher and then to the ambulance for transport. While en route to meet the paramedics, you prepare to start an IV. Considering the patient's present complaint and past medical history, where will you start the IV?

In this chapter, you learn factors that must be considered when locating an appropriate site for IV therapy. Guidelines that further assist you in proper site selection are also presented. At the end of this chapter, we return to this case and apply our knowledge.

QUESTIONS

1. What IV fluid would you use for this patient?
2. What action would you take if the blood vessel you palpated for IV access had a pulse to it?
3. What may happen if you were to start the IV and administer fluid into the patient's left arm?

■ INTRODUCTION

When starting an IV, finding an appropriate site is one of the most important actions you will take. It can often be the difference between successfully or unsuccessfully placing the IV catheter into the vein. Proper site selection is also critical to the overall effectiveness of IV therapy. For instance, if a patient requires a large amount of fluid delivered as quickly as possible, finding a site with large veins, as opposed to small veins, is crucial. Selecting an appropriate site will help avoid complications that can arise if the patient has certain

On Target

Selecting the most appropriate site is a critical step in providing safe and effective IV therapy.

medical conditions or illnesses. The general approach the EMT should take regarding an IV line placement is to make the first attempt the best attempt.

Selecting a Site

On Target

If a patient requires the quick administration of a large volume of fluid, look to the larger veins located in the upper forearm or antecubital fossa. For patients not needing large volumes of fluid, you can use smaller veins found in the lower forearm or hand.

On Target

If a vein for IV therapy is not visible, attempt to locate a vein by palpation.

On Target

Veins should feel "spongy," not hard. Hard structures are most likely tendons or bones, which can be damaged by insertion of the sharp IV catheter.

On Target

If a pulse is felt in a blood vessel, assume it is an artery and do not use it for IV therapy!

When looking for a site to place an IV, begin by asking yourself, "Why am I starting this IV?" If the patient is bleeding, dehydrated, hypotensive, or otherwise requires the quick administration of IV fluids, look for a site with large veins. Large veins can accommodate considerable amounts of fluid, therein allowing rapid placement into the body. Large veins are located in the upper forearm or **antecubital fossa** (**AC**). If the patient does not require large amounts of fluid but is receiving an IV for precautionary reasons or medication administration at a later time, consider smaller veins located on the distal arm or the back (dorsum) of the hand.

Once you have established the need for large or small veins, carefully examine specific areas of the hands or arms that contain the size of vessel required. Look first for veins that are readily visible (techniques for distending veins to make them more visible are discussed in Chapter 6). Veins may be difficult to see if the patient is severely dehydrated, has lost a significant amount of blood, or has large amounts of body fat. In such cases, attempt to locate veins by palpating the area with your fingertips. At times, the best vein to select when attempting an IV is not the most visible one, but the one that is most readily palpable. When palpated, veins have a "spongy" feel to them, not hard. Hard structures are typically tendons or bones, which can be damaged by inappropriate insertion of the sharp IV catheter. Valves within the veins can also feel hard or "knotted." Because valves make placement of an IV difficult, avoid starting an IV in the immediate area. People generally have blood vessels laid out in similar patterns. Familiarity with the "typical" layout of blood vessels can direct you to where veins "should" be. Figures 4.1a and 4.1b show the common locations of veins on the upper arm.

The use of digital palpation with your fingertip can help determine whether there is a vein present that is not readily visible, as well as whether the blood vessel is an artery (which is never used for IV access). When palpating an artery, a pulsation corresponding to each heartbeat can be felt. The lower pressure of blood flowing through the veins does not produce this characteristic pulsation. It is estimated that 10% of the population has some arteries near the surface of the skin, instead of deeper within the skin (as is more common). If a pulsation is felt, assume the vessel is an artery and do not use it for IV access.

It is easier to place an IV into straight veins rather than crooked ones. Look also for **bifurcated veins** (two or more veins coming together to form a single larger vein). Bifurcated veins tend to be well anchored and relatively easy to access (Figure 4.2). Avoid veins that are surrounded by bruised or scarred tissue. Such veins may be damaged, thus not allowing IV fluid to easily flow through them. Also, bear in mind that starting an IV on the underside of the arm tends to be more painful than starting one on the top of the arm.

There may be times when a large vein is necessary for rapid fluid administration but cannot be located or successfully accessed. In such cases,

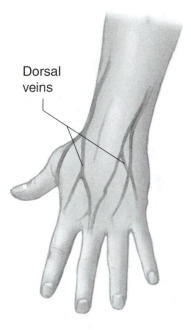

Figure 4.1a. Common peripheral locations of veins used for IV cannulation.

Dorsal veins

it is best to establish the IV in a smaller vein, if available. An IV in a small vein is better than no IV, especially for the critically ill or injured patient. The EMT, paramedic, ALS health care provider, or hospital personnel can make additional attempts for a larger vein at a later time. Although it is appropriate to use the larger veins in the AC for patients requiring fluid

Figure 4.1b. Specific sites of the forearm used for IV cannulation.

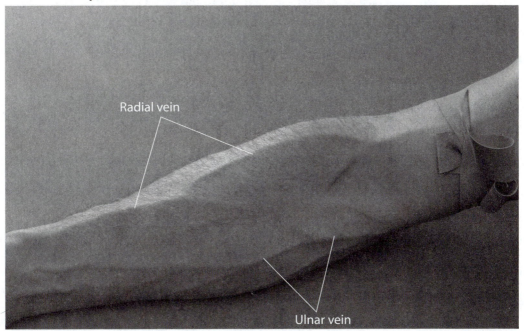

Radial vein

Ulnar vein

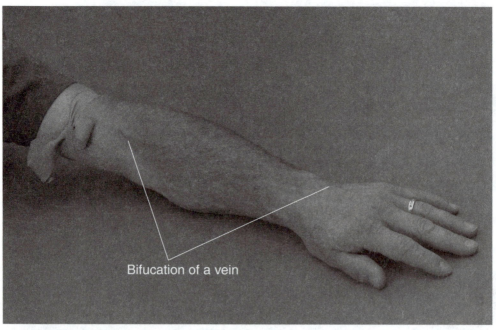

Figure 4.2. Bifurcations in the veins of the arms are often easy to cannulate because they are well anchored and usually larger.

On Target

Remember when establishing an IV in the wrist or antecubital fossa, the IV catheter can become kinked when the patient moves these joints.

volume, it is not necessarily appropriate to use these veins for patients not requiring fluid volume.

Unsuccessful attempts in the antecubital region can damage the blood vessel(s), as well as impair the flow of IV fluids or medication from an IV established at a later time distal to the AC. Therefore, if large amounts of fluid are not required, it is best to start at the hand and work your way up the arm until a suitable vein is located.

When starting an IV around the AC or wrist (joint location), consider that flexion of these joints can "kink" the IV catheter and impair the flow of IV fluid into the patient. Therefore, it is best to start the IV just above or below these joints, not directly over top. Consider whether the patient is right or left handed, and when possible, start the IV in their nondominant side. This permits greater mobility for tasks such as writing and eating. However, in an emergency, this is of minimal concern.

Sites to Avoid

There are certain conditions that prohibit you from using a particular site or even the entire extremity. Using a site when it is inappropriate can result in complications to the patient and/or ineffective IV therapy. These conditions include the following and are summarized in Table 4.1:

- **Dysfunctional or Impaired Arm.** Patients suffering from a stroke or other neurological disease may experience paralysis, weakness, or loss of feeling in an arm. If at all possible, an IV should not be placed in the affected arm.

Table 4.1. Medical Conditions That May Preclude the EMT From Starting an IV in the Immediate Area or Extremity

- Dysfunctional or impaired arm
- Mastectomy (on same arm as side of mastectomy)
- Dialysis shunt
- Skin abnormalities
- Traumatic injuries
- Torturous veins
- Previously used or injured vein
- Swelling

- **Mastectomy (Breast Removal).** If a patient has had a **mastectomy,** avoid placing the IV in the hand or arm on the same side of the body which the breast was removed. The removal of a breast may also involve surgical changes to the circulatory and lymphatic vessels in the same area. Therefore, IV fluids administered into the hand or arm on the same side as the mastectomy may collect in the tissues, resulting in a painful and swollen extremity. If both breasts have been removed, contact medical direction for advisement.

- **Dialysis Shunt.** Persons with chronic renal (kidney) failure often have a dialysis shunt in one arm. A **dialysis shunt** is a surgically placed device that allows the patient to be attached to a dialysis machine (Figure 4.3). Never place an IV in the same arm as the dialysis shunt or in the dialysis shunt itself! Doing so risks physical injury to the shunt and the formation of blood clots or damage from infection. If dialysis shunts are located in both arms, contact medical direction for advisement.

- **Skin Abnormalities.** Because insertion of an IV catheter can introduce foreign material or pathogens (disease-causing agents such as bacteria or viruses) into the body, the IV should not be established in an area

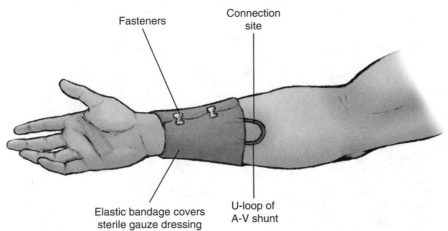

Fasteners

Connection site

Elastic bandage covers sterile gauze dressing

U-loop of A-V shunt

Figure 4.3.
Example of a dialysis shunt found on patients who receive regular dialysis. This site can never be used for IV cannulation.

containing any type of skin disorder. Skin disorders include rashes, abrasions, infections, and burns.

- **Traumatic Injury.** Avoid starting an IV below a site of injury. Injuries such as bone fractures, dislocations, and lacerations can also disrupt the blood vessels in the extremity. If an IV is started below the site of injury, the IV fluids may leak from the vessels, resulting in additional pain and swelling. Always start an IV proximal to the site of injury. If both arms have been traumatically injured, contact medical direction for advisement.

- **Torturous Veins.** Torturous veins are veins that are very angled and/or constantly changing direction. Although the IV catheter is flexible, it cannot make sharp turns or accommodate the sudden bends in such a vessel. Insertion of the sharp IV catheter into a torturous vein can damage the vessel and make it useless for IV therapy. As such, torturous veins should be avoided (Figure 4.4).

- **Previously Used or Injured Vein.** Do not start an IV in an injured vein or in one previously used for IV access. In this instance, "previous" describes a site that was unsuccessfully cannulated during the initial IV attempt. Injured or previously used veins may be damaged and allow IV fluids to escape from the vessel, resulting in localized swelling and pain. If you must restart an IV, find a new site proximal to the previous attempt. Working in a distal to proximal manner prevents IV fluid from having to flow through a vein that is potentially damaged from previous access.

Figure 4.4. **Avoid torturous veins when selecting an IV cannulation site.**

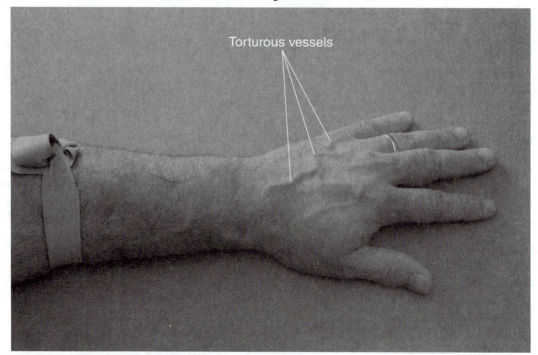

- **Swelling (Edema).** Avoid starting an IV in an area that is swollen. Swelling, or **edema,** is caused by the accumulation of fluid in injured tissues. The fluid can compress veins and impair the flow of IV fluids into the patient, as well as be quite painful. In addition, if the IV fluid leaks from the vein, the amount of swelling and pain will increase. If the swelling is localized, look above the immediate area for a more suitable site or consider the other arm. If both arms are swollen, contact medical direction for advisement.

Enrichment

Some EMS systems may allow the EMT to start an IV in a patient's neck, leg, or scalp. Usually, this is permitted only if there are no sites in the arm available for the IV. Even if not permitted to start an IV in the external jugular vein of the neck, leg, or scalp, familiarity is important because you may perform an interfacility transport of a patient with an IV in any of these areas or be called on to assist an ALS provider who is authorized to establish such an IV.

External Jugular Veins

The neck contains two large veins called the **external jugular (EJ) veins** (one on each side). Because the EJ veins connect directly to larger veins in the trunk of the body, they are well suited for rapid administration of fluids and medications into the central circulation. Establishing an IV in the EJ veins can be difficult and is prone to more complications than an IV in the hand or arm. Do not establish an IV in the EJ vein unless local protocol permits. Generally (but not exclusively), EJ veins are most commonly used for patients in cardiac arrest or who are unresponsive and in critical condition. Figures 4.5a and 4.5b show the location of the EJ vein and an example of an IV established at this site.

Veins of the Lower Extremity

Peripheral veins in the lower legs and feet can also be used for IV access. However, a higher incidence of complications, including infection and the formation of blood clots, has been reported. Blood clots are of particular concern because they can break free and travel to the lungs. A blood clot(s) in the lungs is called a pulmonary embolism and can be fatal. Consequently, most authorities recommend avoiding the legs and feet for IV therapy if at all possible. Never start an IV in the legs or feet unless local protocol permits. Figure 4.6 shows the location of the saphenous vein of the leg and other veins that may be available should the use of the leg be necessary.

Scalp Veins

Scalp veins are sometimes used for IV access in infants. Because placing an IV in the scalp is time consuming and difficult, it is generally reserved for specialized hospital personnel, or for paramedics or nurses with special training. Never attempt to place an IV in an infant's scalp unless specially permitted to do so by local protocol.

On Target

Starting an IV in the external jugular vein, leg, or scalp is more difficult and prone to more complications than an IV started in the arm or hand.

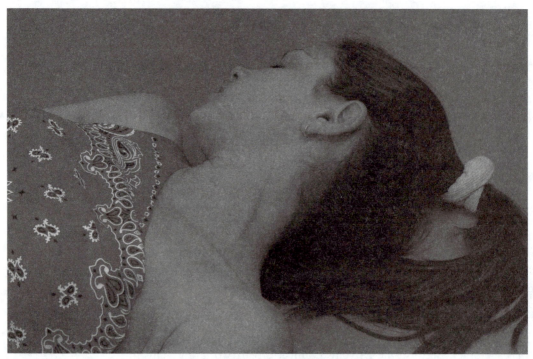

Figure 4.5a. The left external jugular vein in the supine patient.

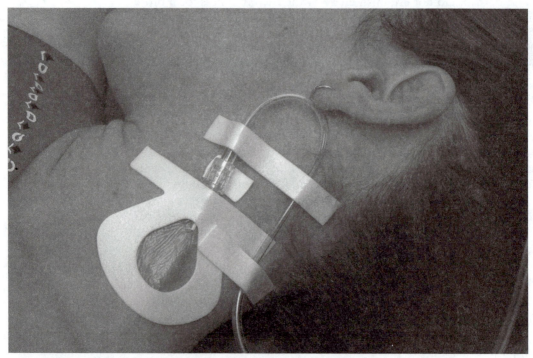

Figure 4.5b. Cannulation of the external jugular vein for IV therapy.

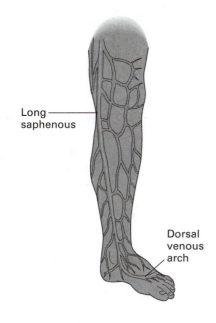

Figure 4.6. **The saphenous vein of the leg can be considered as an IV site, but only as a last resort.**

Long
saphenous

Dorsal
venous
arch

Intraosseous

Intraosseous (IO) cannulation is performed by placing a needle into the medullary cavity (center) of a bone. This is most often done when a pediatric patient needs immediate circulatory access for fluids or medications and a peripheral line cannot be placed (although newer systems have been developed specifically for use in the sternum of the adult). Although placed into a bone, an IO line acts the same as a peripheral venous access site. This skill requires both equipment and technique beyond the scope of this text. For more information, review a critical care or paramedic textbook.

Case Study Follow-Up

You are providing care to a 62-year-old female complaining of general weakness and nausea. After assessing her and providing oxygen, she is moved into the ambulance and transport is initiated. An ALS ambulance with paramedics has been contacted and will rendezvous between the scene and the hospital. The paramedics have asked that you initiate an IV while en route.

While assembling the materials necessary for IV therapy, you consider the most appropriate site to place the IV. Because the patient does not require the rapid administration of fluid, you decide that a smaller vein will be suitable. Because she has a history of breast cancer, you inquire as to whether a breast was removed. The patient informs you that she had part of her left breast surgically removed 2 years ago and that the cancer has not returned. Recognizing a potential complication if the IV is started in the left arm, you examine the right hand and distal right arm for a suitable site.

After applying a constricting band to the patient's right arm, you do not see an obvious vein for access and begin to palpate the back of her hand for a "spongy" feel indicating an underlying blood vessel. You locate a vessel via palpation, and note no pulsation or nearby valves. The skin overlying the vein appears free of swelling and conditions that would preclude use of this site. Knowing that you have located an appropriate site, you successfully establish the IV.

Once you rendezvous with the paramedics, they reassess the patient and attach her to the cardiac monitoring. The paramedics thank you for starting the IV, and the remainder of the transport is uneventful. Later, you find that the patient was admitted to the hospital with an inner ear infection and that the IV was used in the emergency department to administer a medication for nausea.

■ SUMMARY

Choosing an appropriate site for IV placement is a critical step in the delivery of IV therapy. Locating an appropriate site involves more than finding an accessible vein. It is also dependent on the EMT recognizing the reason underlying the IV therapy, along with assessing for specific medical conditions that may preclude a site or entire extremity from being used. Using a site or extremity that is inappropriate may cause complications and/or jeopardize the effectiveness of the IV therapy. The ability of the EMT to successful provide IV therapy may also be called into question. Consequently, it is important that the EMT be knowledgeable of the factors and guidelines used to select an appropriate site for IV therapy.

REVIEW QUESTIONS

1. The most common site used for IV therapy is
   A. arms.
   B. legs.
   C. scalp.
   D. external jugular.

2. You are starting an IV on a patient who requires a large amount of IV fluid delivered very quickly. Which of the following sites contains the most appropriately sized blood vessels?
   A. Antecubital fossa
   B. Leg
   C. Wrist
   D. Hand

3. You cannot see any veins on the arms of a 57-year-old male who is severely dehydrated. You next action would be to
   A. look for a visible scalp vein.
   B. avoid IV therapy.
   C. palpate the hands and arms for potential veins.
   D. start a central IV line.

4. A patient requiring IV therapy has a dialysis shunt in his left arm. Which of the following would be most appropriate?
   A. Place the IV into the dialysis shunt.
   B. Start the IV below the dialysis shunt.
   C. Place the IV in the opposite arm.
   D. Start the IV in a leg vein.

5. You feel a "spongy" blood vessel that pulsates with each beat of the heart. You would
   A. place the IV in the vessel.
   B. look for a new blood vessel.
   C. start the IV just above the pulsation.
   D. press firmly on the vessel to stop the pulsation prior to placing the IV.

6. For prehospital IV therapy, it is *always* best to start the IV in the antecubital fossa.
   A. True
   B. False

7. When starting an IV in a vein located in the wrist area, which of the following statements is true?
   A. The wrist contains the largest veins in the arm.
   B. Flexion of the wrist can impede the flow of IV fluids into the patient.
   C. The wrist contains arteries, not veins.
   D. Tendons in the wrist can be used for IV therapy.

8. It is acceptable to start an IV in the affected arm of a stroke patient.
   A. True
   B. False

9. A patient that requires an IV informs you that she has had a right side mastectomy. Your next action would be to
   A. start the IV on the right side above the mastectomy.
   B. start the IV in the left leg.
   C. look to the left arm for an IV site.
   D. do not start an IV.

10. Placing an IV in an area that is swollen is not advised because it can
    A. increase the amount of swelling.
    B. impede the flow of IV fluid into the patient.
    C. cause an increased amount of pain.
    D. all of the above may result when an IV is placed in a swollen area.

11. You were unsuccessful at placing an IV in the left wrist of a patient with chest pain. What site would be most appropriate to reattempt the IV?
    A. The same site
    B. Left arm
    C. Left hand
    D. Left external jugular vein

12. It is best to use a vein that you can see, rather than one that is more appropriate, but requires palpation to locate.
    A. True
    B. False

13. Which vein runs along the lateral (thumb side) aspect of the forearm?
    A. Cephalic
    B. Basilic
    C. Cephalad
    D. None of the above

14. The external jugular vein is located
    A. inferior to the clavicles.
    B. anterior to the voicebox.
    C. posterior to the carotid arteries.
    D. lateral to the sternocleidomastoid muscle.

15. The most common reason to cannulate the EJ vein is when
    A. the patient is in cardiac arrest.
    B. attempts at using the forearm have failed.
    C. the patient is complaining of chest pain.
    D. the patient is immobilized to a backboard.

Equipment Used for Intravenous Access

LEARNING OBJECTIVES

By the end of this chapter, you should be able to:

- ☑ Identify and describe the different components of macrodrip and microdrip IV tubing
- ☑ Describe the drop factor of IV tubing and relate it to milliliters of IV fluid
- ☑ Identify an over-the-needle IV catheter and describe its different parts
- ☑ Differentiate an over-the-needle IV catheter and a hollow-needle IV catheter
- ☑ Relate the gauge of an IV catheter to its diameter
- ☑ State the importance of not contaminating IV equipment once removed from its packaging
- ☑ Identify the necessary pieces of miscellaneous equipment needed to start an IV and describe their functions

KEY TERMS

Adjustable IV administration tubing—IV administration tubing containing a dial that can be adjusted to various flow rates (number of drops per minute).

Blood tubing—IV tubing used specifically for the administration of blood or blood products.

Drop factor—A specific number assigned to IV tubing that indicates the number of drops that make up 1 milliliter of IV solution.

Extension tubing—IV tubing used to extend or lengthen the original IV administration tubing.

Gauge—A number used to describe the diameter of an IV catheter.

gtt—Medical abbreviation for "drop."

gtts—Medical abbreviation for "drops."

Hollow-needle catheter—An IV catheter consisting of a hollow metal stylet that is inserted into the vein. Hollow-needle catheters are commonly referred to as "winged," "butterfly," or "scalp vein" catheters.

IV administration tubing—IV tubing that allows the delivery of IV fluids to the patient by connecting the IV fluid bag to the IV catheter.

IV catheter—A semiflexible hollow catheter that is placed into the vein. The proximal end has a "female" adapter that couples with the "male" end of the IV administration tubing.

IV tubing—See IV administration tubing.

Macrodrip administration tubing—IV tubing used to rapidly administer large amounts of IV fluid. Macrodrip administration tubing typically divides each milliliter of IV solution into 10, 15, or 20 drops.

Mechanical pump tubing—IV administration tubing used with a mechanical infusion pump.

Measured volume administration set—IV administration tubing containing a burette chamber, which allows precise volumes of IV fluid to be administered.

Microdrip administration tubing—IV administration tubing used to administer small amounts of fluid or to restrict the overall fluid a patient will receive. Microdrip administration tubing typically divides each milliliter of solution into 60 drops.

Over-the-needle catheter—An IV catheter consisting of a semiflexible catheter over top a sharp metal stylet (needle).

Venipuncture device—Sharp needlelike devices used to puncture the patient's skin and access his or her vein.

Venous constricting band—An elastic band used to distend veins by impeding the flow of venous blood once applied to the patient's extremity.

Case Study

You and an EMT student who you are precepting are assessing a 28-year-old male patient who is confused and weak. His airway is patent and his breathing is adequate. His radial pulse is rapid and weak, his skin is cool to the touch, and the conjunctiva of the eyes is dehydrated. The patient's vital signs are pulse, 124 beats per minute; breathing, 18 breaths per minute; and blood pressure, 102/72 mm Hg. He informs you that he has been nauseated and vomiting over the past week, and has had little to eat or drink.

Recognizing that the patient is dehydrated, you instruct your student that she will need to start an IV. She is nervous, so you tell her to prepare the patient for the IV while you gather the necessary materials. Looking into the medical supply bag, you see various items related to IV therapy. Given the patient's condition, what will you select?

Chapter 5 presents the different materials and supplies necessary for IV therapy, as well as the information needed to use them correctly. At the end of the chapter, we return to this case and apply your knowledge.

QUESTIONS

1. Given the presentation of the patient, where on the patient would you most likely start the IV?
2. How would you know the patient has received enough IV fluid and is improving?
3. What would you do if you could not successfully place an 18 or larger gauge catheter into the patient?

■ INTRODUCTION

Establishing an IV requires various materials and supplies. Because you will have to select among and match these items to the needs of the patient, familiarity is essential. Failure to use the appropriate materials for IV therapy may result in undertreatment, overtreatment, or failed attempts—all of which are undesirable. Therefore, it is essential that you have an understanding of the different supplies and materials related to IV therapy, along with the specific indications for their use.

Types of Intravenous Administration Sets

Macrodrip and Microdrip Administration Tubing. **IV administration tubing,** commonly referred to as **IV tubing,** connects the IV fluid bag to the **IV catheter** that is inserted into the patient's vein (discussed later in this section). This permits IV fluid to flow from the IV fluid bag into the patient.

Although there are several types of IV tubing, "macrodrip" and "microdrip" administration tubing are most commonly used in the prehospital setting. **Macrodrip administration tubing** is used when the patient must quickly receive large amounts of IV fluid (e.g., a patient who is hypotensive, dehydrated, or in shock). **Microdrip administration tubing** is used to administer small amounts of fluid and is indicated when the overall fluid a patient will receive must be restricted. Although there are subtle differences between macrodrip and microdrip tubing, they contain many identical parts (Figure 5.1). For illustrative purposes, each part of the tubing is identified and discussed as follows (starting at the proximal end of the tubing and moving distally):

- **Spike.** The spike end of the administration set is a hollow but sharp-pointed plastic device that is inserted into the administration set port

On Target

Macrodrip tubing is indicated for the patient needing rapid administration of large amounts of fluid. Microdrip tubing is best suited for the patient who does not need much fluid or for whom the overall amount of fluid administered must be limited.

Figure 5.1. Note that the only structural difference between microdrip and macrodrip tubing is the drop former. All other components are the same.

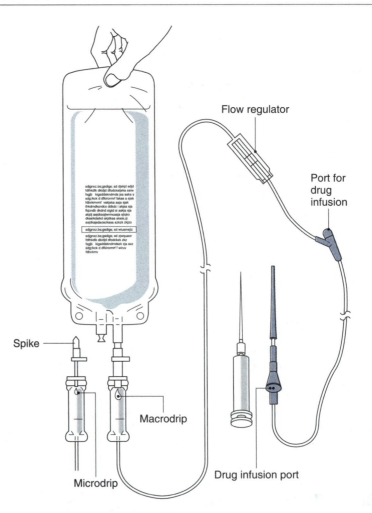

Flow regulator

Port for drug infusion

Spike

Macrodrip

Microdrip

Drug infusion port

on the IV fluid bag. (See Chapter 4 for a description of the administration set port.) Once the spike is inserted into the IV bag, IV fluid can flow from the bag into the administration tubing. The spike is kept sterile by a removable plastic sheath. Once the sheath is removed, you must not touch it or allow it to become contaminated by any means. Failure to keep the spike clean can introduce pathogens (disease-causing agents) into the tubing or IV fluid and into the patient, predisposing him or her to an infection. If at any time the spike becomes contaminated, discard the IV tubing and restart with a new set.

- **Drip Chamber.** The drip chamber is a clear plastic chamber that allows you to view the IV flow rate (Figure 5-1). The flow rate describes the number of drops (**gtts**) of IV fluid (per minute) that flow from the IV fluid bag into the administration tubing and onto the patient. Flow rates are an important aspect of IV therapy that are discussed in greater detail in Chapter 8. The drip chamber is compressible, and when squeezed and released, causes the fluid from the IV bag to accumulate in the clear drip chamber. For proper IV therapy, the drip chamber should always be one-third full of IV fluid. A line on the drip chamber marks this level.

- **Drop Former.** The drop former is located in the drip chamber and transforms the IV fluid in the bag to drops as it enters the chamber itself. The drop former for microdrip tubing is a hollow metal stylet, whereas the drop former for macrodrip tubing is a large plastic circular opening at the top of the drip chamber. Subsequently, the drops formed in microdrip tubing are smaller (*micro,* small), whereas the drops formed in macrodrop tubing are larger (*macro,* large).

Knowledge of the drop former and its operation is important because it is used to calculate precise volumes of fluid. Drop formers are precisely calibrated and assigned a number called the **drop factor.** Although microdrip tubing has a standard drop factor, macrodrip tubing usually comes in three different drop factor settings. The common drop factors for macrodrip and microdrip tubing are as follows:

IV Tubing	Drop Factor	Significance
Microdrip	60	60 gtts = 1 mL of IV fluid
Macrodrip	10	10 gtts = 1 mL of IV fluid
Macrodrip	15	15 gtts = 1 mL of IV fluid
Macrodrip	20	20 gtts = 1 mL of IV fluid

The drop factor allows you to calculate precise fluid volumes by counting drops. For every 60 drops of IV fluid administered with microdrip tubing, 1 milliliter of solution will be delivered to the patient. For every 10 drops of IV solution administered with macrodrip tubing, 1 milliliter of solution will be delivered. (As indicated, macrodrip tubing can also come with drop factors of 15 gtts per milliliter and 20 gtts per milliliter calibrations.) The drop factor is printed on the package containing the IV tubing, as well as on the tubing itself. You must know the calibration of the drop former to calculate flow rates (discussed in Chapter 8).

- **Tubing.** IV administration tubing is clear and flexible (see Figure 5-1). This allows you to monitor the IV fluid as it flows through the tubing, as well as angle and turn it in tight situations. Once the fluid leaves the drip chamber, it travels through the tubing to the patient.
- **Flow Regulator.** The flow regulator is a rolling dial enclosed in a plastic casing (see Figure 5-1). The flow regulator allows you to control the flow rate (rate at which IV fluids are administered to the patient). Flow rates range from wide open (continuous stream) to completely stopped. Rolling the dial toward the IV fluid bag increases the drip frequency and flow of IV fluid into the patient. Rolling the dial toward the patient decreases the drip frequency and slows the delivery of IV fluid. The location of the flow regulator may vary because it can be moved up and down the tubing, but it is found *after* the drip chamber. Although this

is the most common type of flow regulator used prior to hospitalization, another type that allows the EMT to select a specific number of drops per minute does exist and may be used in some systems. It is the EMT's responsibility to become familiar with the specific type of flow regulator used in his or her system.

- **Clamp.** IV tubing has a simple plastic clamp that will stop the flow of IV fluid to the patient when slid over the tubing. The clamp also prevents the entrainment of air into the tubing when changing IV bags (discussed in Chapter 10), as well as the backflow of medication if an advanced care provider administers a drug through the IV after it has been established. The clamp is also useful in stopping the infusion of IV fluid without disturbing the position of the flow regulator.

- **Medication Injection Ports.** Medication injection ports allow medications to be administered through the IV. Some medication ports have a self-sealing membrane into which the hypodermic needle of a syringe containing the drug can be inserted. Other medication ports are "needleless" and will accept a syringe (containing medication) without a hypodermic needle.

- **Needle Adapter.** The needle adapter is located at the distal end of the administration tubing and is designed to fit into the hub of the IV catheter (discussed next). This is commonly referred to as the "male" end of the IV tubing, which is subsequently inserted into the "female" end, or hub, of the IV catheter (discussed next). Similar to the spike, the needle adapter is sterile and covered by a protective cap. If it becomes contaminated at any time, restart with a new administration set.

Venipuncture Devices

Venipuncture describes accessing a patient's vein for IV therapy (*veni*, vein; *puncture*, access into). **Venipuncture devices** are sharp, needlelike devices used to puncture the patient's skin and access his or her vein. There are three basic types of venipuncture devices:

- Over-the-needle catheter
- Hollow-needle catheter
- Plastic catheter inserted through a hollow needle

Over-the-Needle Catheter. The **over-the-needle catheter** (often called an angiocatheter) is the most commonly used venipuncture device in the prehospital setting and consists of a semiflexible IV catheter over top of a sharp metal stylet (needle) (Figure 5.2). There are four parts to an over-the-needle catheter:

- **Metal stylet (needle).** The sharp metal stylet permits easy puncturing of the skin and vein. The stylet is hollow, thus enabling blood from the vein to flow back through the stylet and collect in the flashback chamber (discussed next). The presence of blood in the flashback chamber indicates that the metal stylet has entered a blood vessel.

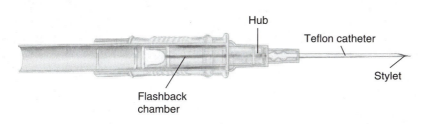

Figure 5.2.
Parts of a typical over-the-needle catheter design used in prehospital care.

- **Flashback chamber.** The clear plastic flashback chamber allows you to see blood after the metal stylet has entered the vein. The presence of blood in the flashback chamber indicates that the metal stylet has entered a blood vessel.

- **IV catheter.** The catheter is a semiflexible hollow tube that resides over the metal stylet. After the metal stylet has punctured the vein, the catheter is slid over the stylet into the blood vessel. This remains in the patient's vein for the duration of the IV therapy or until the IV site must be changed.

- **Hub.** The hub is located on the back of the catheter (female end) and receives the needle adapter (male end) from the IV tubing (after the catheter is removed from the metal stylet). After the IV administration tubing is attached to the hub of the catheter, IV fluid can flow from the fluid bag into the patient.

To prevent the EMT from being accidentally stuck, most over-the-needle catheters contain a spring-loaded mechanism that retracts the sharp metal stylet into the plastic casing of the venipuncture device once the IV catheter has been slid into the vein and the sharp metal stylet has been withdrawn from the patient. It is the responsibility of the EMS provider to become familiar with the type of over-the-needle catheter used within his or her system.

Hollow-needle catheter. For pediatrics or other patients with tiny, delicate veins, a **hollow-needle catheter** may be required (Figure 5.3). Hollow-needle catheters do not have a catheter; rather, the hollow metal stylet itself is inserted into the vein and secured. Because the sharp metal stylet can easily damage the vein, extreme care must be used when establishing an IV with a hollow-needle catheter. Some

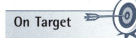

On Target

Over-the-needle catheters are the most commonly used venipuncture device used for prehospital IV therapy.

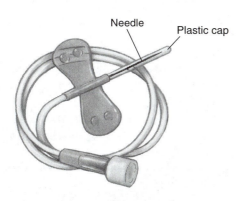

Figure 5.3. **A hollow needle or "winged" catheter set.**

Figure 5.4.
Example of a through-the-needle catheter. These are used when establishing central line catheters in the hospital setting.

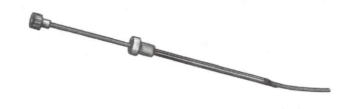

hollow-needle catheters have wings that provide guidance into the vein, as well as a means to secure the catheter after it is in place. Hollow-needle catheters are frequently referred to as "winged," "butterfly," or "scalp vein" catheters. The name "scalp vein" catheter comes from the fact that this is the IV catheter commonly used to initiate an IV in the scalp of a newborn or young infant.

Catheter inserted through the needle. The catheter inserted through the needle (also called an intracatheter) consists of a catheter inserted through a large metal stylet (Figure 5.4). This catheter is used for central IV lines (established in a hospital) and not used in a prehospital setting. Basic familiarity is important because you may be involved in a critical care transport of a patient with a central line established with a catheter inserted through the needle.

Sizing of Intravenous Catheters

IV catheters come in various sizes. The diameter of an IV catheter is expressed as its **gauge.** The larger the gauge number, the smaller the diameter of the catheter and/or stylet. For example, a 22-gauge catheter is smaller than a 14-gauge catheter. Larger-diameter catheters, such as a 14-gauge catheter, allow fluids to be administered more rapidly than smaller-diameter catheters, such as a 22-gauge catheter. It is critical that you consider the reason for starting the IV and choose the appropriate size IV catheter. Indications for the different gauge catheters include the following:

- **22 gauge and 24 gauge.** These extremely small-gauge catheters are indicated for fragile veins such as those of the elderly or pediatric patient.

- **20 gauge.** This small-gauge catheter is best suited for the average adult who does not need immediate fluid replacement. Twenty-gauge catheters are useful when the patient requires IV medications.

- **18 gauge.** The 18-gauge catheter is commonly used for routine IV access. Fluids and/or IV medications can easily be administered through an 18-gauge catheter. Although some authorities consider the 18-gauge catheter to be appropriate for fluid-depleted patients, placement of a larger catheter should be considered.

- **14 gauge and 16 gauge.** The 14- and 16-gauge catheters are large catheters particularly useful for the rapid administration of fluid volume (e.g., shock, hypotension, severe dehydration). A 14- or 16-gauge catheter is indicated when there is a real or potential need for the administration of large amounts of fluid or blood.

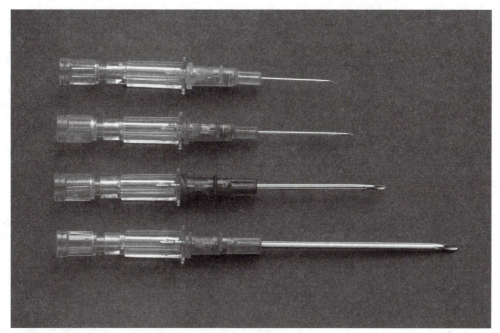

Figure 5.5. **Various IV catheters used in prehospital care.**

Refer to Figure 5.5 for various IV catheter sizes.

Another important characteristic of an IV catheter is its length. Typically the longer the catheter, the greater the resistance to the movement of IV fluid through it, resulting in a slower flow of IV fluid into the patient. Consequently, if the patient requires the rapid administration of a large volume of IV fluid, a short-length (and large-gauge) catheter should be selected. The length of the catheter is rarely a concern when initiating an IV for the purpose of administering medications, unless the short length makes placement well into the vein doubtful.

Table 5.1 shows common equipment utilization given various types of equipment available for IV therapy.

On Target

Use large-gauge IV catheters for the patient requiring the rapid administration of large amounts of IV fluid and smaller-gauge IV catheters when starting an IV on patients not requiring fluid therapy.

On Target

The longer the length of the IV catheter, the slower the flow of IV fluid through it.

Table 5.1. **Equipment Utilization for Intravenous Therapy**

Purpose of IV	Fluid Type	Administration Set	Angiocatheter Size
Fluid replacement from dehydration	RL or NSS	Macrodrip	14–18 gauge
Fluid replacement from blood loss	NSS	Macrodrip or blood administration set	14–16 gauge
Medication administration	NSS or D$_5$W	Microdrip	18–20 gauge

Miscellaneous Equipment

In addition to the IV tubing and catheter, you will need other supplies and materials that include the following:

- **Gloves.** Like any other aspect of emergency care, an IV should never be initiated without protective examination gloves. Because most exam gloves are made from latex, it is important to determine whether the patient has a latex allergy. If the patient or the provider is allergic to latex, nonlatex exam gloves must be used. The same holds true for the venous constricting band, discussed next.

- **Venous Constricting Band.** The **venous constricting band** is an elastic band that is applied proximal to (above) the intended puncture site. When properly applied, the venous constricting band impedes the flow of venous blood, causing the veins to become distended. Distended veins are easier to see and puncture with the venipuncture device. The venous constricting band should never be applied so tightly that it impedes arterial blood flow, nor should it be left in place for more than 2 minutes.

- **Alcohol or Betadine Preparations.** Because IV therapy involves puncturing the skin, there is the potential for pathogens (disease-causing agents) residing on the skin to enter the body and cause an infection. Therefore, it is critical that you use antiseptic preparations such as alcohol or betadine to clean the skin in the area where the IV will be started. Some EMS systems use a combination of both antiseptic agents to help ensure a properly prepared site.

- **Materials to Secure the IV.** After establishing the IV, it must be secured to prevent dislodgment and loss of access. Medical tape is an effective way to secure the IV catheter to the skin and the IV tubing to the patient's arm (discussed in greater detail in Chapter 8). The site where the IV catheter enters the skin must also be covered with a sterile dressing to prevent pathogens from infecting the area. Special membranes designed to cover the site where the IV enters the skin are available. Band-Aid® strips or gauze can also be used to protect the site.

- **Gauze.** Sterile gauze should be on hand for hemorrhage control if you are unsuccessful in establishing the IV or if blood leaks from around the site.

- **IV Prep Kits.** The IV prep kit contains most of the supplies and materials needed to start an IV (IV prep kits do not contain the venipuncture device, IV administration tubing, or IV fluid). Items typically found in IV prep kits are as follows:
  - Antiseptic pads (alcohol and/or betadine)
  - Constricting band
  - Sterile 2 × 2-inch pad
  - Tegaderm® or Veni-guards® for securing the IV puncture site with a sterile cover

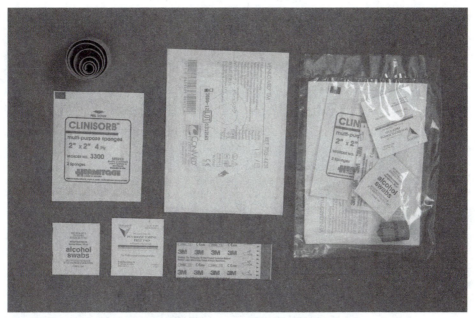

Figure 5.6. Common equipment used when establishing IV access.

Figure 5.6 shows the additional material needed for establishing an IV line beyond that of the IV fluid, IV administration set, and venipuncture device.

Enrichment

In addition to macrodrip and microdrip administration tubing, there are other types of IV tubing that are indicated in certain situations. These include the following:

- IV extension tubing
- Mechanical pump tubing
- Measured volume administration set
- Blood tubing
- Volume-controlled administration tubing

IV Extension Tubing

Extension tubing is IV tubing used to extend or lengthen the original macrodrip or microdrip administration set (Figure 5.7). Like other IV administration tubing, extension tubing is sterile and must be handled accordingly. Extension tubing contains parts similar to macrodrip and microdrip tubing.

Extension tubing allows you to easily change between different types of administration tubing after the IV has been started. For example, if you

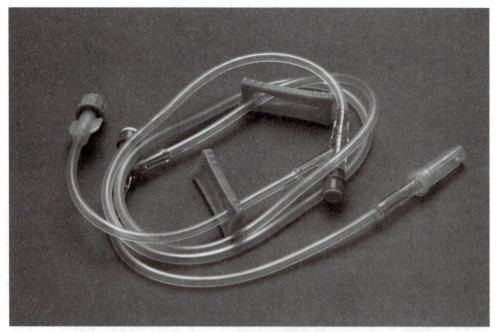

Figure 5.7. Extension tubing is used when additional length is needed for the IV administration set.

must switch from a macrodrip to a microdrip administration set, the clamp on the extension can be closed and the macrodrip tubing detached. Once the microdrip tubing has been prepared, the needle adapter can then be placed into the receiving port on the extension tubing and the clamp released. IV therapy can now be resumed without having to painfully restart another IV line. Changing IV tubing with an extension set in place also decreases the risk of air entering the patient's circulatory system or catheter dislodgment.

Mechanical Pump Tubing

Mechanical IV pumps are devices that precisely regulate the flow and amount of IV fluid and IV medication that a patient receives. Mechanical IV pumps require special tubing parts that allow direct attachment to the pump, as well as filters and relief points for the removal of air bubbles if they become lodged in the tubing. Most times, **mechanical pump tubing** can be used to start a standard IV in the field. Starting the IV with pump tubing may be advantageous if the patient will require a mechanical pump for continued IV therapy once in the hospital. Follow local guidelines concerning the use of pump tubing. Figure 5.8 shows one type of mechanical pump tubing.

Measured Volume Administration Set

A **measured volume administration set** is a device that allows the administration of precise volumes of IV fluid. It consists of either micro- or macrodrip tubing, with the addition of a large burette chamber marked in 1.0-milliliter increments (Figure 5.9). To administer a specific volume of

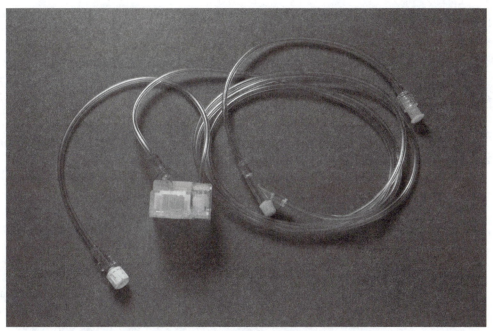

Figure 5.8. **Example of the special administration tubing used with mechanical infusion pumps.**

fluid, the clamp between the IV fluid bag and burette chamber is opened, allowing fluid to drain into the chamber. After the predetermined amount of fluid is in the chamber, the clamp between the IV fluid bag and the burette chamber is closed. The clamp below the burette chamber is then

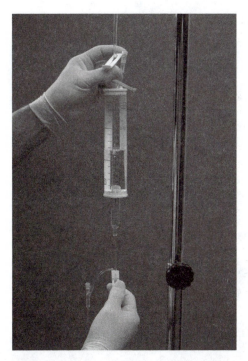

Figure 5.9. **A measured volume administration set.**

opened and the flow regulator adjusted to allow the fluid to be administered at the desired flow rate. After the IV fluid in the burette chamber has been exhausted, you know the exact amount of fluid administered.

Measured volume administration sets are beneficial for patients who need specific or limited volumes of fluid (e.g., pediatrics or other patients with conditions intolerant of fluid overload). The measured volume administration set is also useful for infusing an IV medication that must first be mixed in a specific amount of IV fluid. Basic preparation of a measured volume administration set is discussed in Chapter 6. For more information concerning measured volume administration sets, consult a critical care or paramedic textbook.

Blood Tubing

Blood tubing must be used any time blood or blood components are administered. Because blood that is stored or administered over an extended period is prone to form clots and/or accumulate other debris, it must be filtered during administration. Consequently, blood tubing contains a filter through which the blood must pass prior to entering the patient. Failure to use blood tubing when administering blood may allow blood clots to enter the patient and travel to the blood vessels in the lungs, resulting in a pulmonary embolism (blood clot lodged in a blood vessel in the lungs). A pulmonary embolism can be fatal.

Blood tubing comes in "Y" and "straight" configurations (Figure 5.10). "Y" tubing has two spikes, one for blood and one for IV NSS. Typically, blood is administered with NSS because fluids such as LR increase the potential for damage to the blood (hemolysis). The two-spike design enables the EMT to

Figure 5.10. Blood administration sets may be designed as either a "straight" (right) or "Y"(left) type.

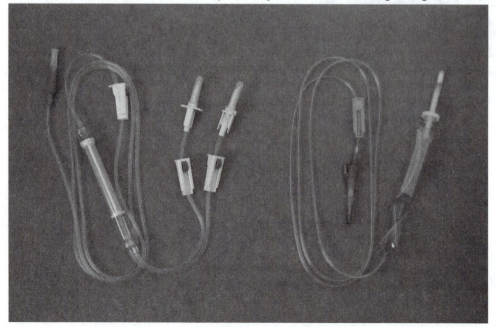

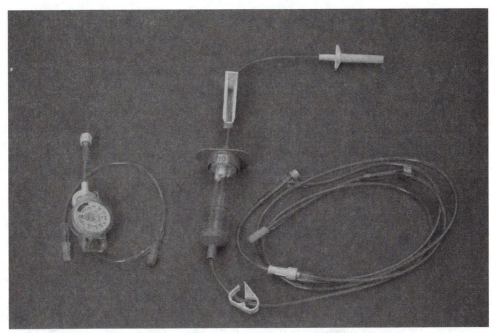

Figure 5.11. Photo of two different styles of adjustable administration sets.

start an IV with blood tubing and hang NSS as he or she would when start-ing other IVs. Once in the hospital or in the presence of other ALS providers capable of administering blood, the blood can be attached to the other spike for immediate administration. If the blood supply is exhausted or must be shut down for any reason, the NSS can then easily be restarted. If "straight" tub-ing is used, only one IV fluid (NSS or blood) can be used at a time.

Although the EMT will probably not administer blood or blood prod-ucts in the field setting, he or she may want to use blood tubing for a patient who has experienced blood loss or otherwise requires blood re-placement. On arrival at the hospital or rendezvous with an ALS provider capable of administering blood, it can be immediately infused without hav-ing to change the IV administration tubing or restart the IV.

Adjustable IV Administration Tubing

Adjustable IV administration tubing contains a dial that adjusts the specific flow rate (number of drops per minute administered). Other IV adminis-tration sets can be adjusted to either microdrip or macrodrip configura-tions (Figure 5.11).

On Target

Consider blood tubing for any critical trauma patient. Although the EMT will not administer blood, having the blood tubing in place on arrival at the hospital saves time because hospital personnel will not have to start another IV using the blood tubing and can administer blood or blood products to the patient without delay.

Case Study Follow-Up

You and the EMT student who you are precepting must start an IV on a 28-year-old dehydrated patient. Because the student is nervous, you instruct her to prepare the patient for IV therapy while you gather the appropriate supplies and materials.

Reaching into the medical supply bag, you select macrodrip IV administration tubing calibrated at 10 gtts per milliliter because this will allow the fast administration of a large amount of IV fluid. Likewise, you select a 16-gauge, over-the-needle catheter to facilitate fast administration of IV fluid. A 1,000-milliliter bag of 0.9% NSS is also chosen. Looking at your student, you see that she has applied the venous constricting band and is ready to start the IV.

Nervously, the student starts the IV and is excited when she sees that her first attempt is successful! After administering the first bag of IV solution, the patient's heart rate comes down to 76 beats per minute and he states that he feels much better. In the emergency department, he is further treated for dehydration, and as a precaution, admitted for 24-hour observation before being released.

■ SUMMARY

Various supplies and materials are available to the EMT for IV therapy. Knowledge of these items is essential because many have specific functions and/or indications for use. Selecting the appropriate equipment allows the EMT to tailor the IV therapy to the particular needs of the patient. Lack of familiarity can result in IV therapy that does not meet the needs of the patient or is otherwise ineffective, and perhaps even dangerous. Therefore, it is the EMT's responsibility to possess a working knowledge of this equipment so proper IV therapy and patient care can be provided.

REVIEW QUESTIONS

1. A hypotensive patient who is severely dehydrated requires the rapid administration of a large amount of IV fluid. Which of the following pieces of IV equipment would be most appropriate?
   A. Microdrip administration tubing
   B. 24-Gauge IV catheter
   C. Macrodrip administration tubing
   D. Microdrip administration tubing with a 14-gauge IV catheter

2. Failure to keep the spike on the IV administration tubing sterile or clean can result in
   A. clogging of the drip chamber.
   B. infection of the patient.
   C. too slow of a flow rate.
   D. clogging of the catheter.

3. You are using IV administration tubing with a drop factor of 10 gtts mL. As such, which of the following is true?
   A. A maximum of 10 drops can be given over 1 minute.
   B. For every 10 drops of IV solution given, the patient's blood volume will increase by 10 mL.

    C. One drop of IV solution equals 10 mL of IV solution.

    D. Ten drops of IV solution equals 1 mL of IV solution.

4. Where would the EMT look to find the drop factor of IV tubing?

    A. Flow regulator

    B. Tape used to secure the IV tubing to the patient

    C. Package containing the IV tubing

    D. IV catheter

5. The function of the flow regulator is to

    A. increase or decrease the flow of IV fluid.

    B. connect the IV fluid bag to the patient.

    C. increase or decrease the drop size of IV fluid.

    D. attach the IV tubing to the IV catheter.

6. Which of the following best describes an over-the-needle venipuncture device?

    A. Hollow needle that does not have a catheter

    B. IV catheter that contains a catheter inserted through a large metal stylet

    C. Catheter over top of a metal stylet

    D. Small IV catheter with "wings"

7. When starting an IV, you notice the presence of blood in the flashback chamber. This would indicate

    A. the metal stylet is in a blood vessel.

    B. the patient requires blood or blood products as an IV solution.

    C. a smaller IV catheter must be used.

    D. IV fluid is moving from the IV fluid bag into the patient.

8. A hollow-needle IV catheter ("butterfly") is best suited for

    A. situations in which large amounts of IV fluid must be delivered.

    B. placement in a large blood vessel.

    C. extremely small veins.

    D. use with a 14-gauge IV catheter.

9. A patient requires IV access, not for fluid but for medication administration. As such, which size IV catheter would be most appropriate?

    A. 12 Gauge

    B. 14 Gauge

    C. 16 Gauge

    D. 20 Gauge

10. For a patient requiring a large amount of IV fluid to be administered very quickly, which of the following would be most appropriate?
    A. 16 Gauge
    B. 20 Gauge
    C. 22 Gauge
    D. 24 Gauge

11. When using a venous constricting band, it is important to
    A. place it above the intended site for IV access.
    B. apply it tight enough to restrict the flow of arterial and venous blood.
    C. leave it in place for 2 minutes after the IV has been established.
    D. apply it tight enough to restrict the flow of arterial blood.

12. Using alcohol or betadine preparations in conjunction with IV therapy is important to
    A. distend veins.
    B. increase the chance for successful placement of an IV.
    C. minimize the opportunity for infection.
    D. distend both veins and arteries.

13. Which of the following IV catheters would be best to quickly administer large amounts of blood to a trauma patient in shock?
    A. 14 Gauge, 1¼ in. in length
    B. 16 Gauge, 2 in. in length
    C. 18 Gauge, 1¼ in. in length
    D. 20 Gauge, 1 in. in length

14. Which of the following is the *best* explanation of why blood should be administered through a blood solution set?
    A. Blood tubing has a microdrip-size drop former.
    B. Blood tubing has an inline filtration system.
    C. Blood tubing has multiple spikes.
    D. Blood tubing does not have medication administration ports.

15. Which calibration is best for the patient requiring limited fluids?
    A. 10 gtts/mL set
    B. 15 gtts/mL set
    C. 20 gtts/mL set
    D. 60 gtts/mL set

Obtaining Intravenous Access

LEARNING OBJECTIVES

By the end of this chapter, you should be able to:

☑ State the importance of cleansing the intended site of puncture with alcohol or betadine preparations

☑ State the importance of taking BSI precautions when starting an IV

☑ Describe the appropriate technique for establishing an IV in the hand or arm

☑ Define flow rate and describe a wide-open (WO) and to keep open (TKO)/keep vein open (KVO) rate

KEY TERMS

Flow rate—Rate at which the IV fluid is administered to the patient.

Keep vein open—A flow rate at which just enough IV fluid is administered to keep the body from forming blood clots at the end of the IV catheter once placed in the vein.

KVO—See Keep vein open.

Pathogens—Microorganisms capable of causing disease.

TKO—See To keep open.

To keep open—A flow rate at which just enough IV fluid is administered to keep the body from forming blood clots at the end of the IV catheter once placed in the vein.

Wide open—A flow rate in which IV fluid is administered freely to the patient.

WO—See Wide open.

Case Study

The medical director for your EMS service requires all EMTs to perform 8 hours of clinical time each month with him in the emergency department. During your rotation, the medical director asks you to help assess a geriatric patient from a long-term care facility who is being evaluated for a change in mental status.

At the patient's side, the medical director instructs you to assess the patient as you would in the field setting. At the completion of your assessment, the medical director states that he is impressed and shows you a few advanced techniques that build on your existing assessment skills. He continues by asking what you would do for this patient in the field. You reply that among other interventions, you would start an IV in the patient. The physician agrees and instructs you to do so now. Furthermore, he wants to observe your technique while you explain the rationale for each step. How will you proceed?

In Chapter 6, you learn the technique necessary to properly place an IV. Flow rates, or the rate at which IV fluids are administered to the patient, are also presented and discussed. At the end of this chapter, we return to this case and apply your knowledge.

QUESTIONS

1. Would a 14- or 16-gauge IV catheter be appropriate for this patient?
2. How is a TKO rate of benefit to this patient?
3. Why use a hand vein for the IV and not the AC, where the veins are larger and generally easier to access?

■ INTRODUCTION

When establishing an IV, it is critical that you use proper technique by performing specific actions in a certain order. Doing so will allow you to become proficient when starting IVs and will increase the likelihood of successful placement, while decreasing the opportunity for complications that can accompany IV therapy.

Infection Control

On Target

Cleaning the intended puncture site with an alcohol and/or betadine is critical in minimizing the opportunity for infection.

Gaining IV access is an invasive process that breaks the protective barrier of the skin. You must remember that there are **pathogens** (disease-causing agents such as bacteria) on the skin that can be introduced into the body and cause infection unless removed prior to insertion of the IV catheter. Cleaning the intended puncture site with an alcohol and/or betadine is an important measure to help prevent pathogens from gaining entry into the patient's body during the introduction of the needle into the skin. When cleaning the site with alcohol or betadine, start at the intended puncture site and work outward in an expanding circular motion. This will push pathogens away from the puncture site. Failure to do so provides an opportunity for pathogens to enter the body during insertion of the IV catheter, causing a localized or even systemic (bodywide) infection.

Because insertion of an IV catheter involves puncturing into the patient's vein, you may be exposed to blood. Some infectious diseases (e.g., hepatitis, AIDS) can be spread from person to person via contact with infected blood. Therefore, it is best to assume all blood is infectious and take the appropriate BSI precautions. At a minimum, gloves must be worn, and goggles are highly recommended.

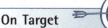

On Target

Because inserting an IV catheter into a patient's veins may expose the EMT to blood, gloves must always be worn. Goggles are highly encouraged!

Establishing an IV in the Hand or Arm

As an EMT, you will most often establish an IV in the hand or arm (what is termed as "peripherally"). The veins of the hands and arms are relatively easy to locate and produce fewer complications than IVs placed in other areas. To establish a peripheral IV in the hand or arm, use the following technique:

1. **Determine the indication for IV therapy.** Start by considering the reason for the IV therapy and select the appropriate equipment. Use macrodrip tubing with a large-diameter IV catheter (14, 16, or 18 gauge) for a patient requiring volume replacement. Consider microdrip tubing or a measured volume control administration set with a smaller-diameter IV catheter (18, 20, or 22 gauge) for any patient whose IV fluid must be restricted or who requires IV access for medication administration or precautionary reasons. Select the appropriate IV fluid as determined by local medical direction.

2. **Gather and arrange the appropriate supplies and materials.**
   - IV fluid
   - IV administration tubing
   - IV catheter
   - Antiseptic preparation (betadine and/or alcohol)
   - Venous constricting band
   - Tape or commercial securing device

3. **Take BSI precautions.** At a minimum, gloves must be used, and goggles are highly recommended.

4. **Prepare the IV solution bag and IV administration tubing.**
   a. After removing the IV bag from its outer packaging, examine the IV bag for leaks and the fluid for clarity and expiration date. Never use an IV fluid that is cloudy, contains particulate matter, or is expired.
   b. Slide the flow regulator on the administration tubing toward the drip chamber, position it about 1 to 3 inches away from the drip chamber and then close it off completely (rolling the wheel toward the needle adapter).
   c. Remove the protective sheath from the spike on the IV tubing and insert it into the IV fluid bag's administration set port.
   d. Squeeze the drip chamber until the IV fluid reaches the fill line (approximately one-third full).

On Target

Never use an IV fluid that is cloudy or expired. Discard it and select a new fluid.

e. Open the flow regulator to allow the fluid to fill the tubing and expel all air from the line. *Important:* Most IV tubing has a protective cap over the needle adapter at the distal end, which is vented to let the air escape as you flush the line. It is *not* necessary to remove the protective cap and risk contaminating the set. *Only* loosen the cap if fluid *does not* flow through the line readily after opening the flow regulator.

f. Allow the fluid to flow through the administration set until all air and trapped bubbles are eliminated. At this point, the IV line is "primed."

g. Stop the flow of IV fluid through the tubing by closing the flow regulator.

Remember that the IV tubing is sterile. If at any time the spike or needle adapter becomes contaminated, obtain new tubing and start over.

5. **Select the puncture site.** Use the guidelines as discussed in Chapter 4 when selecting the IV site. Good sites have the necessary size veins for therapy and should be free of bruising and/or scarring. Straight veins are easier to access than torturous ones.

6. **Place the venous constricting band.** Place the venous constricting band approximately 2 inches proximal to (above) the intended site of puncture. Apply it tightly enough to impede venous, but not arterial blood flow. Check for a distal pulse *after* applying the constricting band to ensure you have not accidentally blocked the arterial blood flow.

   Avoid placing the venous constricting band over joints or under loose clothing (because it may be forgotten if not visible). Never leave the constricting band in place for more than 2 minutes.

7. **Cleanse the intended puncture site of pathogens.** Using alcohol and/or betadine preparations, start at the intended puncture site and work outward in an expanding circle. After cleansing the site, *nothing* can touch the intended puncture site. Do not repalpate the site with your fingers or clean the tip of your finger with alcohol and then touch the site. If you should need to recleanse the site, do so, but never with previously used alcohol. Some EMS systems have the EMS providers use both alcohol and betadine to prepare the skin prior to placing the IV. Be sure to follow the protocol established by the medical director.

On Target

To ensure the catheter is introduced into the vein, insert the over-the-needle catheter 0.5 cm further into the vein after blood is observed in the flashback container.

8. **Insert the IV catheter into the vein.** With your nondominant hand, pull the local skin taut to stabilize the vein; this helps prevent the vein from rolling. With the bevel of the metal stylet up, insert the needle of the venipuncture device into the vein at a 10- to 30-degree angle. Continue insertion until you feel the catheter "pop" into the vein or see blood in the flashback chamber. The metal stylet is now in the vein; however, the catheter may not. To place the catheter into the vein, carefully advance the device another 0.5 cm further. (Carefully advance the needle itself if using a butterfly catheter that does not have the catheter over the needle.)

9. **Slide the catheter into the vein.** While holding the venipuncture device stationary, slide the catheter off the stylet and into the vein. (Never withdraw the needle from within the catheter and then attempt

to reinsert the needle as this can cause a piece of catheter to shear off into the bloodstream.) Once the catheter is inserted to the hub, place a finger over the vein where the distal end of the catheter resides. Gently press downward to tamponade (occlude) the vein against the tip of the catheter. This prevents blood from flowing out of the catheter and air from entering the circulatory system through the catheter. Carefully remove the metal stylet and immediately discard it in a needle disposal container. Remove the venous constricting band.

10. **Obtain venous blood samples, if indicated.** (Discussed in Chapter 10.)

11. **Attach the IV tubing to the IV catheter.** Remove the protective cap from the needle adapter and tightly secure it into the catheter hub. Ensure the IV is patent by opening the flow regulator and freely administering IV fluid for several seconds. Use the flow regulator to achieve the appropriate flow rate. (Flow rates are discussed next.)

12. **Secure the IV catheter and administration tubing.** Do not let go of the IV catheter and administration tubing until they are secured! Secure the IV catheter by placing tape across the hub. Cover the site with a sterile commercial device, if available. Some EMS systems require the application of an antibiotic ointment over the IV insertion site. Loop the IV tubing to make the medication administration port easily accessible. Secure the tubing to the patient with tape.

13. **Label the IV solution bag.** Write the following information on a label and affix it to the IV fluid bag as required:

    • Date and time initiated

    • Person initiating the IV

    Do not write directly on the fluid bag because the ink may be absorbed through the bag and into the IV fluid.

14. **Continually monitor the IV, flow rate, and the patient for complications.** (Discussed in Chapter 8.)

    See Figures 6.1a through 6.1i.

Flow Rates

The **flow rate** is the rate at which IV fluids are administered to the patient. (Flow rate may also be referred to as the drip rate.) The flow rate at which an IV fluid is delivered can vary from a **wide-open (WO)** to a **to keep open (TKO)** rate. A WO rate describes the rapid administration of IV fluids in which the solution runs freely into the patient. TKO (also referred to as **keep vein open** or **KVO**) is a flow rate in which a minimal amount of fluid is used to keep the blood from clotting at the end of the catheter. If the blood clots at the end of the catheter, the flow of IV fluid into the patient will cease, necessitating reinitiation of the IV. Typically, a TKO rate is the delivery of 1 drop of IV fluid every 3 to 5 seconds. Flow rates can be set anywhere between these two extremes. Monitor the flow rate by observing the frequency of drop formation in the drip chamber. Use the flow regulator as described in Chapter 5 to adjust the flow rate. Medical direction may order a specific flow rate.

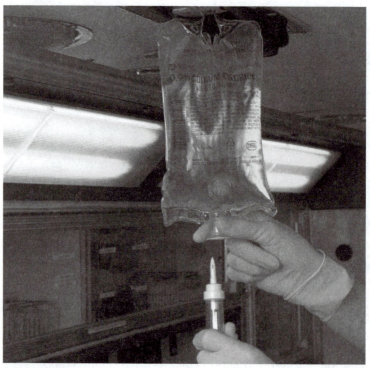

Figure 6.1a. Spike the bag.

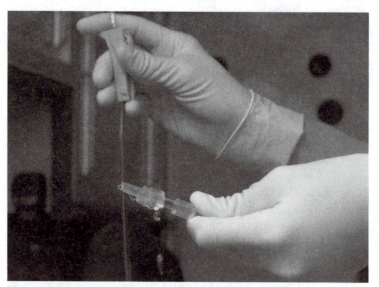

Figure 6.1b. After filling the drip chamber, flush all air from the tubing.

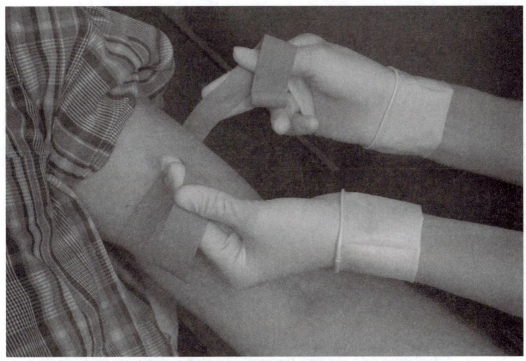

Figure 6.1c. Apply the constricting band above the intended site of cannulation.

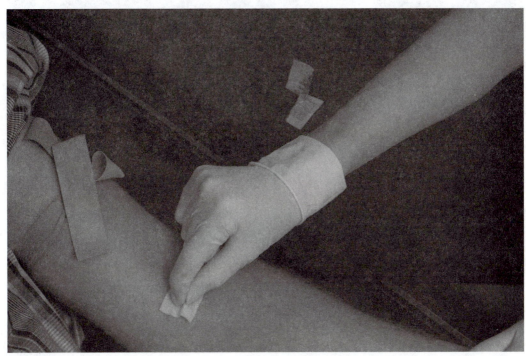

Figure 6.1d. Cleanse the site with an alcohol or betadine prep in a circular motion moving outward.

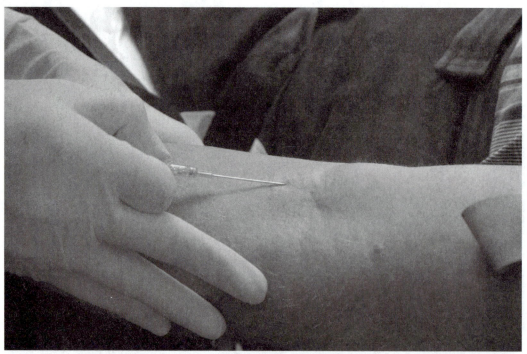

Figure 6.1e. Stabilize the vein, and with the bevel up on the catheter, puncture into the skin.

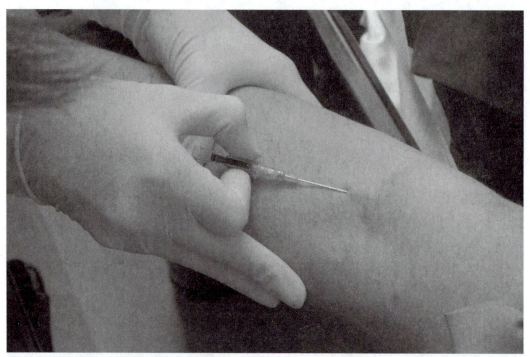

Figure 6.1f. After piercing into the vein, you will notice the sudden loss of resistance ("pop"), and blood will appear in the flashback chamber. Then advance the device another 0.5 cm to place the catheter in the vein.

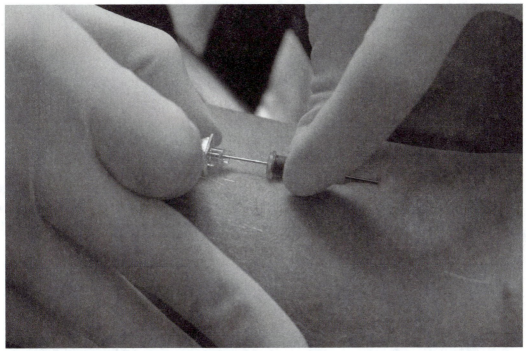

Figure 6.1g. While holding the needle thread the catheter off the needle and into the vein.

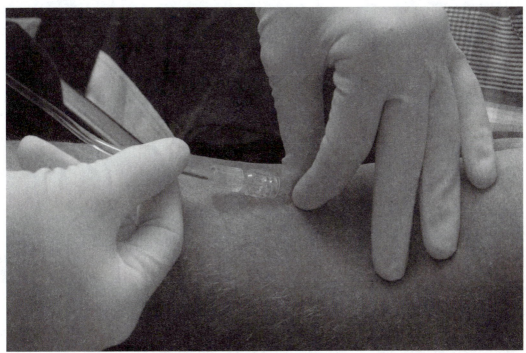

Figure 6.1h. While tamponading the vein, hold the catheter hub still and attach the IV tubing. Be sure not to accidentally contaminate the insertion site.

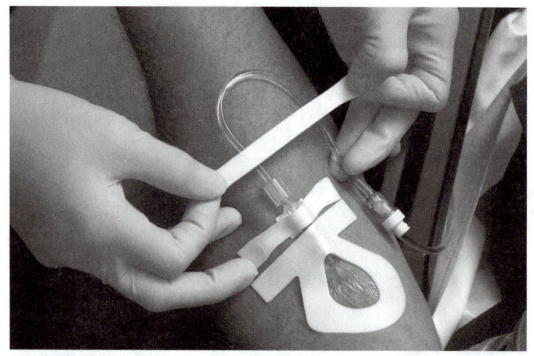

Figure 6.1i. **After ensuring patency, secure the site using appropriate sterile dressings and securing devices.**

Enrichment

Some EMS systems may allow the EMT to start an IV in the external jugular (EJ) vein. The EJ vein is a large peripheral blood vessel in the neck between the angle of the jaw and the middle third of the clavicle. It connects into the subclavian vein of the central circulation. Because the EJ vein lies so close to the central circulation, fluids and medications rapidly reach the core of the body from this site.

The neck and EJ vein is an extremely painful site to access and possesses the opportunity for more complications than the veins in the hands and arms. Therefore, the EJ should be considered for an IV only if the patient is unresponsive or all means of establishing IV access in the hands and/or arms have been exhausted. As always, only use the EJ if local protocol permits.

Accessing the EJ vein requires the same materials as IV access in the hands and arms, plus a 10-milliliter syringe. Because a venous constricting band is never placed on the patient's neck, it is not necessary. Use the following technique when establishing an IV in the EJ vein (Figures 6.2a to 6.2e):

1. **Determine the need for IV therapy, and select the appropriate IV administration tubing and catheter.** Because the EJ is a large vein, larger-diameter IV catheters (14, 16, 18 gauge) and macrodrip tubing are typically used.

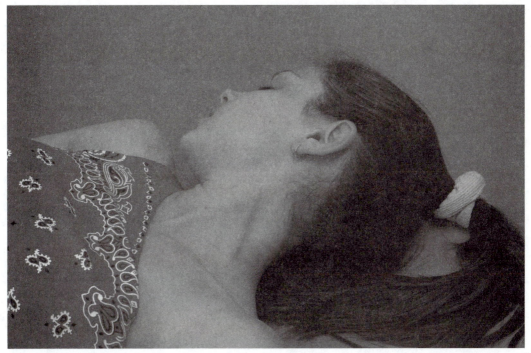

Figure 6.2a. Place the patient in a supine or Trendelenburg position and roll the head opposite of the intended insertion site.

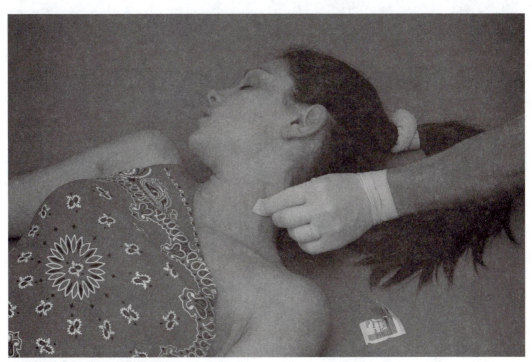

Figure 6.2b. Cleanse the site.

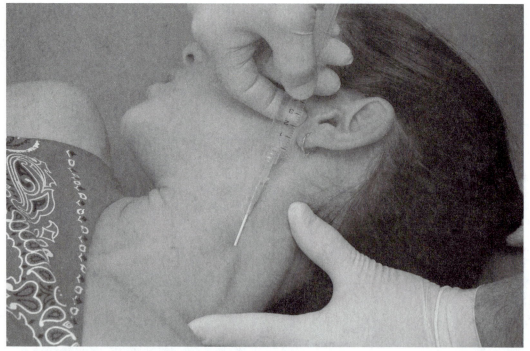

Figure 6.2c. Tamponade the jugular vein distally with your index finger and pierce into the blood vessel while gently aspirating on the saline-filled syringe.

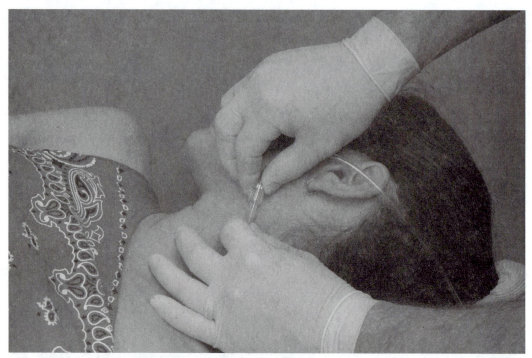

Figure 6.2d. After successfully cannulating the jugular vein, remove the needle and attach the IV tubing. Be sure not to contaminate the site.

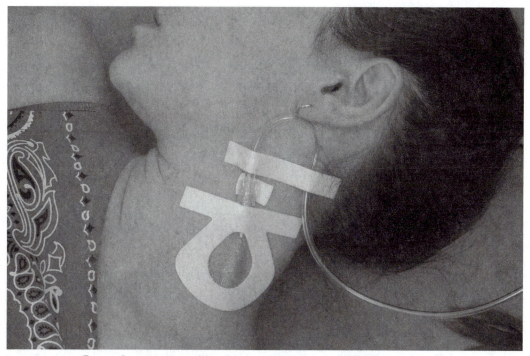

Figure 6.2e. Dress the puncture site with sterile dressings and secure the tubing as appropriate.

2. **Prepare all equipment as for peripheral IV access in the hand or arm.** Some authorities advocate the use of a 10-milliliter syringe when starting an IV in the EJ. If local medical direction permits EMTs to access the EJ and requires use of the 10-milliliter syringe, obtain and fill a 10-milliliter syringe with 3 to 5 milliliters of sterile saline.

3. **Attach the syringe to the flashback chamber of the venipuncture device.**

4. **Take BSI precautions.** At a minimum, gloves must be used, and goggles are highly recommended.

5. **Place the patient supine or in the Trendelenburg position.** Placing the patient supine and/or in the Trendelenburg position increases blood flow into the chest and neck, thus engorging the EJ, making it easier to see and puncture with the IV catheter. The supine or Trendelenburg position also decreases the chance of air entry into the circulatory system during the IV attempt.

6. **Turn the patient's head to the side opposite of access.** By turning the patient's head to the side opposite of the attempt, the EJ is easier to see and puncture with the IV catheter. Do not move the patient's head and neck if a traumatic head or neck injury is suspected.

7. **Cleanse the intended puncture site of pathogens.** Using alcohol and/or betadine preparations, start at the intended puncture site and work outward in an expanding circle.

8. **Occlude venous return by placing a finger on the EJ vein just above the clavicle.** Occlusion as such should distend the vein, assisting in greater

visualization and ease of puncture. Never apply a venous constricting band around the patient's neck!

9. **Insert the IV catheter.** Position and insert the venipuncture device parallel with the vein at bevel up (at a 10- to 30-degree angle) midway between the angle of the jaw clavicle and the medial third of the clavicle.

10. **Withdraw the plunger on the syringe as the venipuncture device enters the EJ vein.** A "pop" should be felt and blood seen in the barrel of the syringe when the IV catheter enters the EJ vein. Once inside the vein, advance the needle another 0.5 cm so the tip of the catheter lies well within the vein.

11. **Slide the catheter into the vein.** Slide the catheter over the stylet into the vein as described for IV access in the hand or arm. Carefully remove the metal stylet and immediately discard it in a needle disposal container.

12. **Obtain venous blood samples, if indicated.** (Discussed in Chapter 10.)

13. **Attach the IV tubing to the IV catheter.** Remove the protective cap from the needle adapter and tightly secure it into the catheter hub. Ensure the IV is patent by opening the flow regulator and freely administering IV fluid for several seconds. Use the flow regulator to achieve the appropriate flow rate.

14. **Secure the IV catheter and administration tubing.** Do not let go of the IV catheter and administration tubing until they are secured. Secure the IV catheter by placing tape across the hub. Cover the site with a commercial device, if available. Use tape to secure the IV tubing to the patient's neck.

15. **Label the IV fluid bag.** Write the following information on a label and affix it to the IV fluid bag as required:

   • Date and time initiated

   • Person initiating the IV

   Do not write directly on the fluid bag because the ink may be absorbed through the bag and into the IV fluid.

On Target

The EJ should only be used if medical direction allows EMTs to establish an IV in this location.

16. **Continually monitor the flow rate and the IV and patient for complications.** (Discussed in Chapter 8.)

Although using the EJ vein has advantages, it also has distinct drawbacks. You may inadvertently puncture the airway or damage nearby arterial vessels. To minimize risks, perform the procedure carefully and never attempt IV access in the EJ unless local medical direction permits.

Intravenous Access Using a Measured Volume Administration Set

If using a measured volume administration set, use the following technique (Figures 6.3a to 6.3d):

1. Prepare the tubing by closing all clamps, and insert the flanged spike into the IV solution bag's spike port.

2. Open the airway handle and the flow control valve between the IV bag and the burette chamber. Fill the burette chamber with approximately 20 milliliters of fluid.

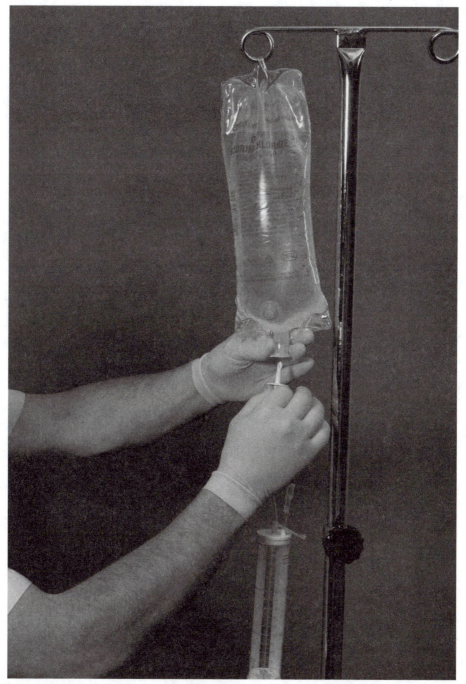

Figure 6.3a. The first step is to close all clamps on the tubing, and then insert the spike into the IV bag.

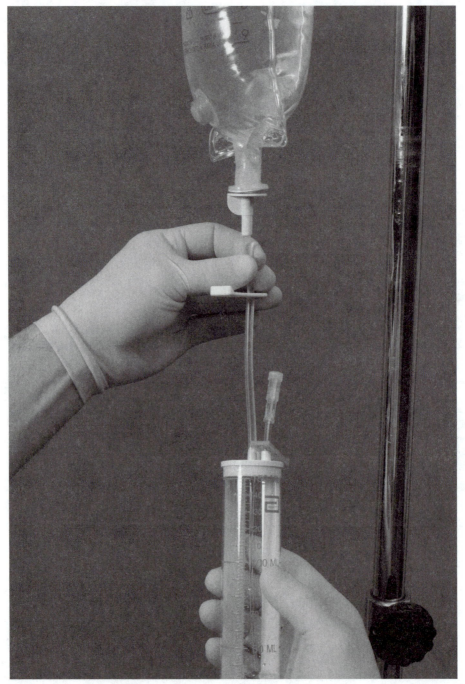

Figure 6.3b. Open the air valve and flow control between the IV bag and the burette chamber to allow the chamber to fill with fluid.

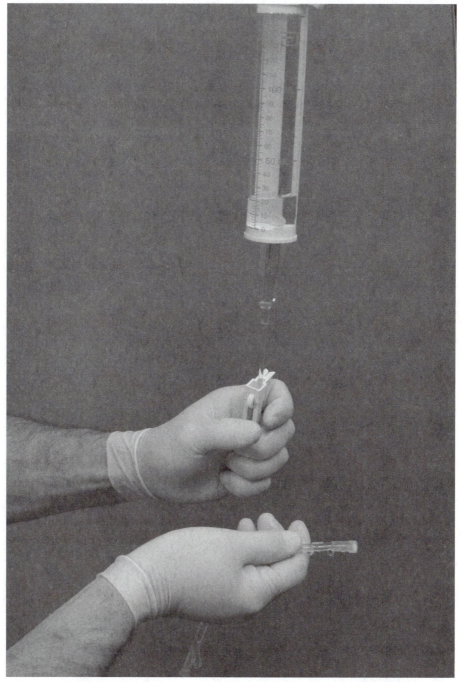

Figure 6.3c. Expel the air from the line by flushing the fluid through. When done, close the **lower flow control.**

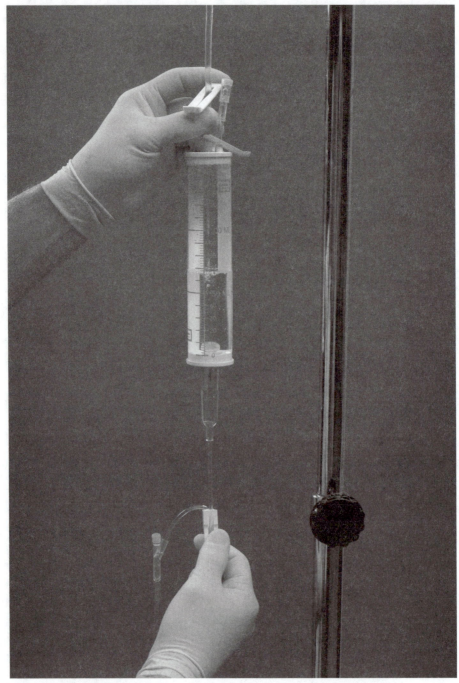

Figure 6.3d. Fill the burette chamber with the desired amount of fluid.

3. Squeeze the drip chamber beneath the burette chamber until the fluid reaches the fill line.

4. Open the bottom flow regulator to prime and purge air from the tubing. When all air is purged, close the bottom flow regulator.

5. Continue to fill the burette chamber with the desired amount of solution.

6. Close the uppermost clamp and open the flow regulator until you reach the desired drip rate. Leave the airway handle open so air replaces the displaced fluid.

To refill the burette chamber, close the clamp on the administration tubing and open the uppermost clamp until the burette chamber is refilled to the desired amount. Release the clamp and continue administration.

You can also use the burette administration tubing for continuous fluid administration. Fill the burette chamber with at least 30 milliliters of solution and close the airway handle. Leave the uppermost clamp open and adjust the rate with the lower flow regulator.

Intravenous Access Using Blood Tubing

If using blood tubing, prepare the administration set using the following procedure (Figures 6.4a to 6.4d):

1. Prepare the tubing by closing all clamps and inserting the spike into the NSS.

2. Squeeze the drip chamber until it is one-third full of NSS.

3. Prime the tubing with NSS.

4. Attach blood tubing to the IV catheter (or into the medication administration port of a previously established IV line).

5. Ensure patency by infusing a small amount of NSS and adjust to the desired flow rate once patency is confirmed.

Hospital personnel or ALS health care providers can now attach a bag of blood or blood components for immediate administration to the patient.

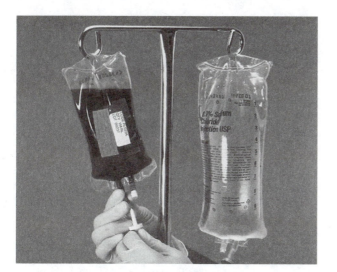

Figure 6.4a.
Insert the spiked end of the blood tubing into the bag. Ensure lower flow control valves are shut off.

Figure 6.4b. Fill the drip chamber as normal.

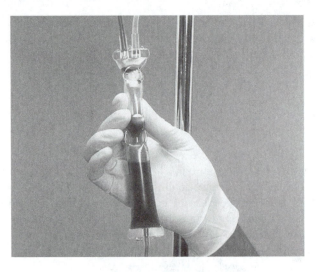

Figure 6.4c. Attach the male end of the blood tubing into the female end of the catheter.

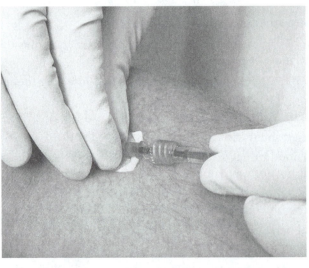

Figure 6.4d. Establish the desired flow rate of the fluid.

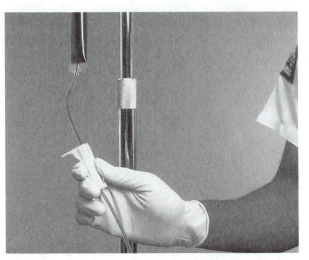

Case Study Follow-Up

You must start an IV in the presence of your medical director. Furthermore, he asks that you explain the rationale for each step as you perform it. While you apply gloves and goggles, a nurse enters the room with the IV fluid bag and administration tubing already prepared.

Finding a potential site on the patient's left hand, you inform the medical director that you are going to apply a venous constricting band above this area to help distend the vein and make it easier to access with the over-the-needle catheter. Because you do not want to introduce pathogens into the patient's body, causing a localized or systemic infection, you clean the site with alcohol and allow it to dry. The physician acknowledges your actions and hands you a 20-gauge, over-the-needle catheter. With your nondominant hand, you pull the patient's skin taut to stabilize the vein and keep it from rolling. You tell the physician that this will make access easier.

With the venipuncture device bevel up, you insert it into the vein at a low angle. You explain that the presence of blood in the flash-back chamber indicates that the needle is in the vein, but advance it a little further to ensure the catheter is also in the vein. After sliding the catheter over the needle into the vein, you press down on the vein over the area where the tip of the catheter lies to prevent air from entering the patient's circulatory system and blood from flowing out of the catheter. The sharp metal stylet is removed and promptly disposed of in the needle container at bedside.

Removing the protective cap from the IV administration tubing, you connect it to the hub of the catheter and open the flow regulator to allow several milliliters of IV fluid to run freely into the patient. Because the patient is not fluid depleted, you inform the physician that a TKO flow rate is adequate. Accordingly, you adjust the flow rate so 1 drop is administered every 5 seconds. Stating that you are still concerned about infection, you place a protective membrane over the IV site and secure the tubing to the patient's arm with medical tape. You finish by labeling the IV bag with the appropriate information.

Your medical director is so impressed with all of your actions and technique that he lets you go home early after only completing 4 hours of your rotation. On your way out, the nurse informs you that you must complete the appropriate IV documentation sheets. As you complete them, you notice that the patient is your medical director's mother.

■ SUMMARY

Although starting an IV is not difficult, it does demand that the EMT use proper technique and perform a series of steps in the appropriate order. Doing so will not only increase your chance of successfully placing an IV, but it will also minimize the opportunity for complications that can arise from IV therapy. (Specific complications are discussed in Chapter 7.) Taking measures to prevent infection of both patient and provider is an important aspect of IV therapy. Accordingly, the EMT must always take the appropriate BSI precautions and ensure the IV puncture site has been cleaned prior to insertion of the venipuncture device and protected after the IV has been established. Promptly disposing of the sharp needle stylet in the proper container or using venipuncture devices equipped with a protective sheath are critical because accidental needle sticks remain a significant cause of health care-related injuries.

REVIEW QUESTIONS

1. Cleaning the intended site of puncture with alcohol and/or betadine preparations is important because it
   A. makes the skin easier to puncture with the venipuncture device.
   B. allows the EMT to skip the application of a venous constricting band.
   C. causes the vein to distend and become easier to access.
   D. removes and pushes pathogens away from the intended site of puncture.

2. What is the minimal BSI precaution that should be taken by the provider when starting an IV?
   A. Gloves
   B. Goggles
   C. Gloves and gown
   D. Gloves, goggles, and gown

3. The IV administration tubing is fully prepared or "primed" when
   A. the tubing is filled with IV fluid and all air bubbles are eliminated.
   B. the drip chamber is completely full.
   C. the tubing is connected to the hub of the IV catheter and fluid is flowing into the patient.
   D. the flow regulator is open but the IV fluid does not come out of the tubing.

4. A venous constricting band has been properly placed when
   A. over top of a joint.
   B. tight enough to impair the flow of venous blood.
   C. below the intended puncture site.
   D. taut enough to impede both venous and arterial blood flow.

5. When cleaning a puncture site with alcohol, the EMT should

   A. pour a minimum of 5 ounces of alcohol over the site and let it dry.

   B. cleanse the site with soap and water, followed by alcohol.

   C. start at the intended puncture site and work outward in an expanding circular motion.

   D. wipe the site with an alcohol preparation using a horizontal stroke for a minimum of 30 seconds.

6. When puncturing the skin with a venipuncture device, the EMT should

   A. enter the skin with the bevel up at a 10- to 30-degree angle.

   B. insert the venipuncture device with the bevel down at a 45-degree angle.

   C. enter the skin at a 90-degree angle until blood is observed in the flashback chamber.

   D. insert the venipuncture device at a 15-degree angle with the bevel down.

7. When starting an IV, you observe blood beginning to enter the flashback chamber. Your next step would be to

   A. attach the administration tubing to the hub of the IV catheter.

   B. close the flow regulator.

   C. close the flow regulator and slide clamps.

   D. advance the venipuncture device slightly further into the vein.

8. You have just placed an IV catheter into a vein and attached the administration tubing. IV fluid flows freely into the patient, and the proper flow rate is obtained. Your next step would be to

   A. secure the IV catheter and tubing with medical tape.

   B. slide the catheter off the needle stylet.

   C. fill the drip chamber to the appropriate level.

   D. label the IV with the appropriate information.

9. A flow rate is described as

   A. the size of the drop formed in the drip chamber.

   B. the rate at which the blood forms clots at the end of the IV catheter.

   C. the configuration of IV administration tubing and size of the venipuncture device.

   D. the rate at which IV fluids are administered to the patient.

10. A physician orders you to administer IV fluids to a patient at a WO rate. You would

   A. provide one drop every 10 seconds.

   B. open the flow regulator so IV fluid passes freely into the drip chamber.

    C. administer 100 mL of solution and then stop the flow of all IV fluid.

    D. attach the IV fluid bag directly to the hub of the IV catheter.

11. A TKO or KVO rate is best described as
    A. one drop every 3 to 5 seconds.
    B. administering 100 mL of IV fluid over 10 minutes.
    C. one drop every 10 to 20 seconds.
    D. freely administering the entire bag of IV fluid.

Factors Affecting Flow Rate and Complications of IV Therapy

LEARNING OBJECTIVES

By the end of this chapter, you should be able to:

- ☑ Identify factors and conditions that can impede the flow of IV fluid into the patient
- ☑ Describe the specific actions taken to rectify any factor or condition that impedes the flow of IV fluid into the patient
- ☑ Describe complications that may result from IV therapy
- ☑ Describe measures necessary to prevent and manage specific complications from IV therapy

KEY TERMS

Anticoagulant—Medication that "thins" the blood, making it more difficult to clot.

Air embolism—Air bubbles that enter the patient's circulatory system.

Edema—Swelling caused by the collection of fluid in interstitial areas of the tissues.

Extravasation—Condition in which IV fluid escapes from the vein and collect in the surrounding tissues.

Hematoma—Collection of blood underneath the skin.

Infiltration—A complication of IV therapy in which the vein has been punctured more than once and IV fluid is allowed to escape into the surrounding tissues.

Necrosis—Formation and shedding of dead tissue.

Pulmonary embolism—A blood clot lodged in the blood vessels of the lungs.

Pyrogenic reaction—A complication caused by pyrogens that enter the body when establishing the IV. A pyrogenic reaction is characterized by the abrupt onset of fever (100°F to 106°F), chills, backache, headache, nausea, and vomiting.

Pyrogens—Microorganisms or foreign proteins capable of producing a pyrogenic reaction.

Thrombophlebitis—A condition in which the vein becomes inflamed.

Thrombus—Blood clot.

Case Study

You have just arrived as back-up on the scene of a motor vehicle collision with multiple patients. The triage officer directs you to a 26-year-old male patient who is still being extricated from the car in which he was trapped. The report given to you was that he was an unrestrained driver traveling at a high rate of speed prior to hitting a tree. The patient struck the steering column and is currently complaining of chest and abdominal pain. After being extricated by the fire department onto a backboard, you note that the IV started while he was still entrapped is no longer flowing properly. How will you determine what is wrong?

In Chapter 7, you learn about factors and conditions that affect the flow of IV fluids into the patient. General complications associated with properly and improperly established IVs are also presented. Techniques for managing and correcting these factors, conditions, and complications are discussed. At the end of the chapter, we return to this case and apply your knowledge.

QUESTIONS

1. When restarting the IV on this patient, what type of IV administration tubing would you use?
2. How do you know that the problem with the IV is infiltration and not a locally infected site?
3. What has happened to the vein to cause it to infiltrate?

■ INTRODUCTION

Your responsibility for the IV does not end after it has been established. You must ensure the IV is flowing properly while monitoring the patient for any related complications. Various complications can arise secondary to even properly performed IV therapy, whereas a host of various other factors and conditions can impede the flow of IV fluid into the patient. You must be able to assess for factors or conditions that can hinder the flow of IV fluids into the patient, along with any complications that may originate secondary to the IV therapy. Once a problem is identified, the appropriate corrective action must be taken.

Factors Affecting the Flow of IV Fluids into the Patient

A patent IV allows IV fluid to easily flow into the patient at the desired flow rate. Sometimes, the IV will not run properly (even if started with proper technique), as evidenced by the slow to nonexistent movement of IV fluid through the drip chamber despite the flow regulator being in a WO position. There are several reasons why an IV might not flow properly—some minor reasons requiring a simple action to correct and some major reasons requiring that the IV be restarted in another location. If the IV fluid fails to run at a satisfactory rate, you must identify the problem. Look for any of the following:

- **Venous Constricting Band Left in Place.** Ensure the venous constricting band has been removed. Because the constricting band compresses the vein and slows the movement of blood to the core of the body, the flow of IV fluid into the patient will also be hindered. If the constricting band is still in place, remove it and look to the drip chamber for improvement in the flow rate. Similarly, tight-fitting clothing or an inflated blood pressure cuff above the IV catheter can interfere with the flow of IV fluids.

- **Infiltration and Extravasation.** A vein is considered infiltrated when it has been punctured more than once, which causes the IV fluid being infused to escape the vessel and collect in the surrounding tissues. **Infiltration** is most often the result of accidentally inserting the IV needle too far into the vein, causing it to puncture the posterior wall of the vessel. Similarly, threading the catheter too forcefully into the vein can cause it to puncture the vessel more than once, resulting in infiltration. Infiltration can also occur if the distal tip of the IV catheter lies outside the vein instead of inside it.

  Extravasation is the medical term that describes IV fluid that has collected outside the veins (*extra,* beyond; *vasation,* blood vessel). If you notice a poor flow rate along with **edema** (swelling) and/or a **hematoma** (collection of blood under the skin) just above the insertion site, suspect infiltration and extravasation of the IV fluid. The patient may also complain of pain at the IV site.

  An infiltrated IV is not usable and must be restarted above the present site or in the other extremity. Figure 7.1 depicts what an infiltrated IV would appear like with associated extravasation of fluid.

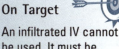

On Target

An infiltrated IV cannot be used. It must be removed and restarted.

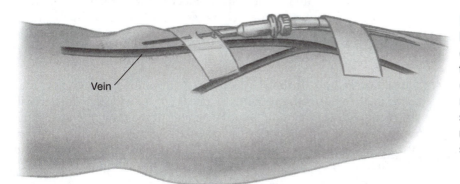

Vein

Figure 7.1.
Extravasation of fluid can occur when the tip of the catheter is outside the vein. This results in a slowing and stoppage of flow. There may also be pain and swelling at the site.

Figure 7.2. **If the tip of the catheter is against a valve, the flow may become unreliable.**

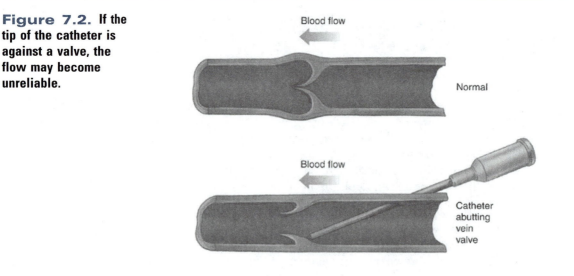

Blood flow

Normal

Blood flow

Catheter abutting vein valve

On Target

When repositioning the IV catheter, the EMT must be careful not to pull it out of the vein.

- **Catheter Tip Abutting the Vein Wall or Valve.** If the distal tip of the catheter lies against the wall or valve of a vein, the flow of IV fluids may be impeded (Figure 7.2). If you believe this to be the case, carefully pull back on the catheter to reposition it. This may require removing tape and retaping the catheter once an adequate flow rate has been achieved. You might also consider using an arm board to stabilize the patient's hand or arm if movement of the extremity causes the catheter to intermittently touch the vein wall or valve.

- **IV Tubing Clamps or Flow Regulator Closed.** Ensure the flow regulator and all clamps of the IV tubing (and IV extension tubing, if used) are open.

- **IV Bag Positioned Too Low.** The proper flow of IV fluids into the patient is dependent on gravity. Therefore, the IV bag must be held/hung well above the site of catheter. An IV fluid bag positioned too low will not flow adequately. As a general rule, the IV bag should be positioned above the patient's head (Figure 7.3).

- **Excessive Fluid in the Drip Chamber.** A drip chamber that is too full will not allow IV fluid to flow freely from the bag into the administration tubing. If the fluid in the drip chamber is above the fill line, invert the IV bag and squeeze the drip chamber so the excess IV fluid is transferred back into the IV bag. Since IV fluid is clear, careful observation of the drip chamber is required to identify if it becomes overfilled (Figures 7.4a to 7.4c).

- **Thrombus at End of the IV Catheter.** A **thrombus** (blood clot) that forms at the end of the catheter or needle of a butterfly catheter will obstruct the flow of IV fluid into the patient. If the flow rate is slowing, use the flow regulator to slightly increase the rate of IV fluid delivery into the patient. This will prevent the formation of a thrombus and keep the IV patent (open). If the flow rate has completely stopped,

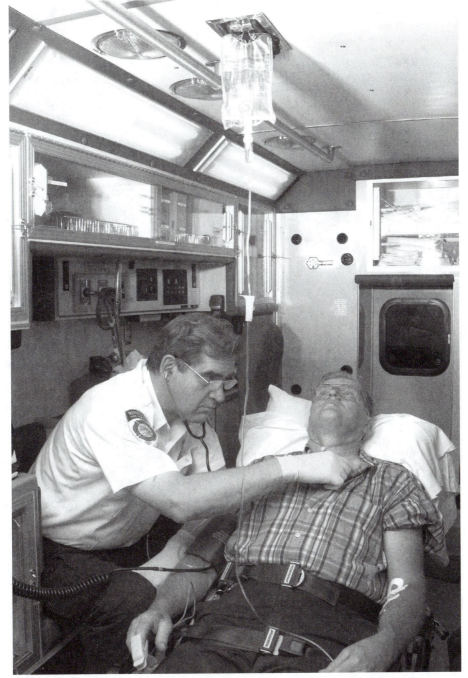

Figure 7.3. Because the IV fluid infuses due to gravity, the IV bag must be positioned at a level higher than the patient.

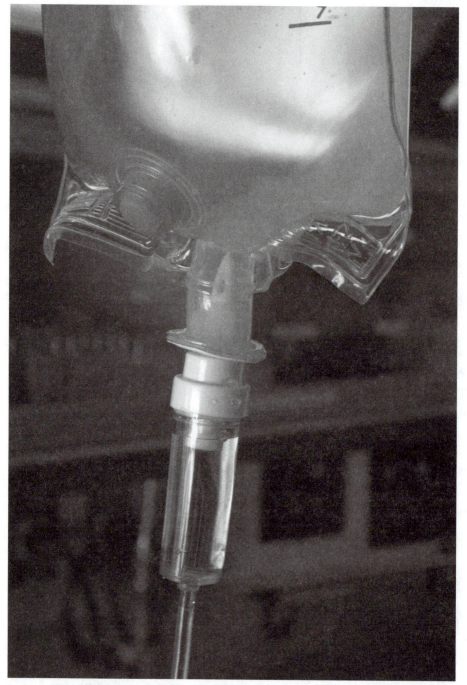

Figure 7.4a. Fluid in the drip chamber is higher than the drop former. This complication must be corrected to ensure good fluid flow.

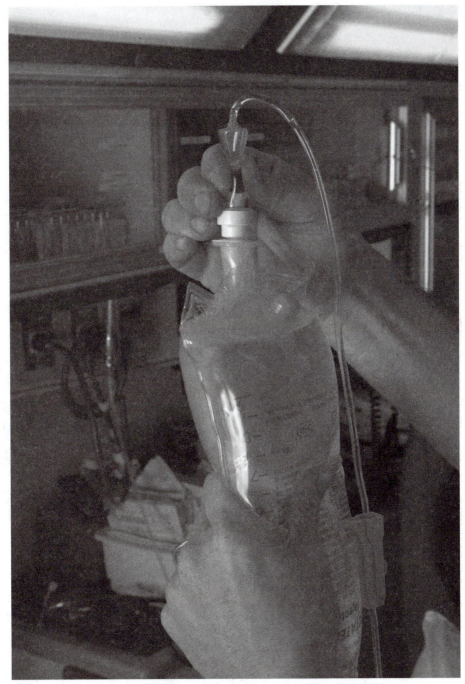

Figure 7.4b. Invert the bag and squeeze the excess fluid back into the IV bag.

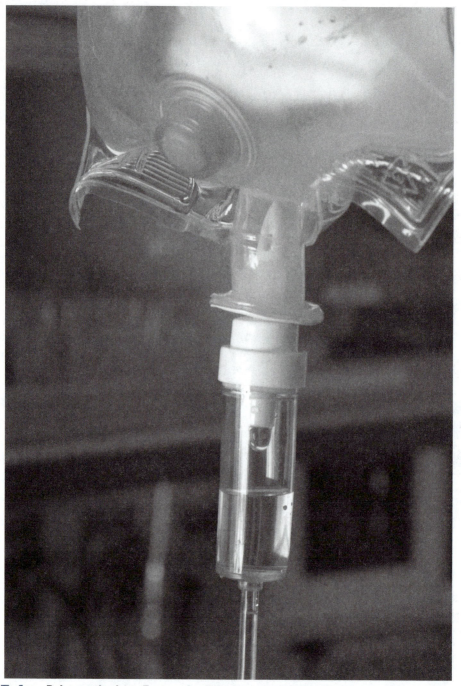

Figure 7.4c. Reinvert the bag. Ensure the flow has returned at the appropriate rate. Repeat this process as needed.

cleanse the medication administration port closest to the IV catheter and attach a syringe. Gently pull back on the plunger of the syringe until the blood is aspirated into the syringe barrel (then discard the syringe into a sharps container). Never fill a syringe with saline and flush an IV that has stopped running. This may dislodge a blood clot, causing it to move through the circulatory system into the lungs, resulting in a pulmonary embolism. A **pulmonary embolism** is a serious medical condition that can cause death.

- **Equipment Malfunction.** An equipment malfunction is an uncommon reason for an IV to cease flowing. When a piece of IV equipment is defective, it should be identified by the EMT as the materials are gathered, checked, and set up. Obtain new materials for any piece of IV equipment that is defective.

  If the IV tubing becomes "kinked," the flow of fluid into the patient will cease. Kinked tubing most often results from patient movement and poor technique in taping the tubing to the patient's arm. Compression of the tubing is another cause of poor fluid movement from the IV fluid bag into the patient. A piece of heavy equipment placed on top of the tubing or tubing that is trapped between a wheel of the cot and the floor of the ambulance are common causes of compression. The EMT should track the course of the IV tubing to ensure it is free from these types of problems.

If flow rate remains poor after considering all these possibilities, move the IV fluid bag below the level of the catheter insertion. If blood flows into the IV administration tubing, the site is patent and the problem lies elsewhere. If blood does not flow into the IV tubing, it must be removed and restarted at another site with new materials. Removal of an IV is discussed in Chapter 10.

Complications of Intravenous Therapy

Although IV therapy is a routine intervention in the prehospital setting, it is not a benign procedure. Numerous complications can accompany even properly performed IV therapy. These complications include the following:

- **Pain.** Pain is common during the insertion of the venipuncture device or when complications such as infiltration and extravasation occur. Occasionally, health care providers apply an anesthetic cream (4% lidocaine cream) to the site where access is intended to reduce the pain associated with starting an IV. However, this practice is uncommon in the prehospital setting because it can take from 30 minutes to 1 hour for the anesthetic to take effect.

- **Local Infection.** If the skin is not thoroughly cleansed with alcohol and/or betadine prior to insertion of the IV catheter or if the equipment is unknowingly contaminated by the EMT, pathogens can enter the patient and cause a localized infection. An infection may also occur if you improperly handle the catheter and allow it to become contaminated

On Target

Never fill a syringe with saline and flush an IV that has stopped running. This may dislodge a blood clot and cause a pulmonary embolism.

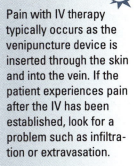

On Target

Pain with IV therapy typically occurs as the venipuncture device is inserted through the skin and into the vein. If the patient experiences pain after the IV has been established, look for a problem such as infiltration or extravasation.

prior to insertion. A localized infection does not occur immediately, but it becomes apparent hours to days after the IV has been placed. Signs of a localized infection include pain at the IV site, as well as tenderness and inflammation. To avoid causing a localized infection, thoroughly cleanse the IV site with alcohol and/or betadine and avoid contaminating the IV catheter prior to use. Covering the IV insertion site after the IV has been established will also prevent infection by limiting the entry of pathogens into the immediate area.

- **Pyrogenic Reaction. Pyrogens** (foreign proteins capable of producing fever) in the administration tubing or IV fluid can cause a **pyrogenic reaction.** Most often, a pyrogenic reaction occurs when the IV fluid is contaminated by a microorganism or other foreign matter. The abrupt onset of fever (100°F to 106°F), chills, backache, headache, nausea, and vomiting characterize a pyrogenic reaction. The vein in which the catheter is placed may also be reddened and painful as the reaction progresses up the arm. In severe cases, death may result. Typically, a pyrogenic reaction occurs ½ to 1 hour after the IV has been initiated.

  Never prepare and assemble an IV at the beginning of the shift for use at a later time. Although this may decrease the time required to set up an IV during a call, it also exposes the IV to pyrogens and other foreign material present in the back of the ambulance. Subsequently, the opportunity for a pyrogenic reaction is greatly increased.

  If you suspect a pyrogenic reaction, immediately discontinue and remove the IV and reestablish it at another site with new materials, including the IV fluid. In addition, bring all the IV equipment with you to the hospital when you deliver the patient. This allows the hospital to examine the IV materials to determine if they are contaminated. Pyrogenic reactions are very serious and underscore the need to discard any IV fluid that is cloudy or any equipment that has been opened (Figure 7.5).

- **Allergic Reaction.** Although a rare occurrence, any patient receiving IV therapy may develop an allergic reaction. Most allergic reactions occur with the administration of blood or colloidal IV solutions; however, most IV administration sets contain latex and may cause a reaction in a patient who is allergic to it.

  The sudden onset of hives (urticaria), itching (puritis), localized or systemic edema, and/or shortness of breath are signs of an allergic reaction. If an allergic reaction is suspected, immediately stop the IV infusion and remove the catheter from the patient. Treat the patient as any other person experiencing an allergic reaction. Use nonlatex materials for any patient who is allergic to latex. Figure 7.6 depicts the skin effects common to an allergic reaction.

- **Catheter Shear.** A catheter shear occurs when the catheter of the over-the-needle catheter is pulled back over the metal stylet after being partially or fully threaded off the metal stylet. The catheter can easily snag on the sharp tip of the metal stylet and shear off, thus forming a plastic emboli. The emboli can enter the circulatory system and lodge in the blood vessels of the lungs, causing a pulmonary embolism. Therefore,

On Target

Always ask the patient about an allergy to latex. If the patient is allergic, use nonlatex IV materials and gloves.

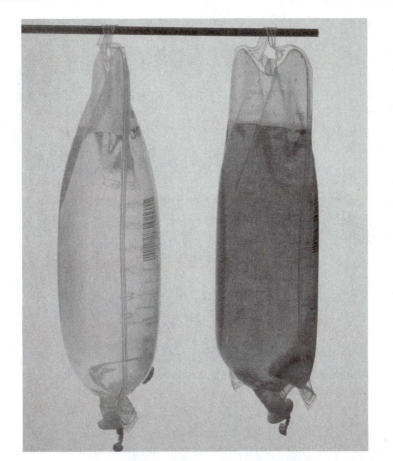

Figure 7.5. IV fluids used prehospital should always appear clear. If cloudiness or discoloration is noted, do not use the IV bag.

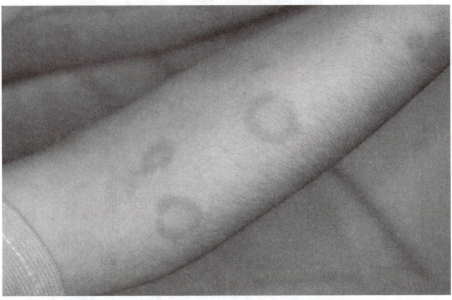

Figure 7.6. Skin findings of hives and redness that correspond to an allergic reaction. This may be seen in susceptible patients during IV initiation or fluid administration.

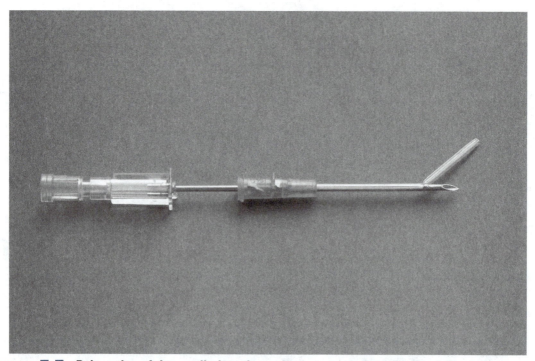

Figure 7.7. Reinsertion of the needle into the catheter may result in the tip of the catheter shearing off and lodging elsewhere in the body.

it is critical that you never pull the catheter back over the metal stylet after both have been inserted into the vein. Figure 7.7 shows how a catheter shear could occur.

On Target

To avoid placing an IV in an artery, palpate the blood vessel in which you are attempting the IV. If the vessel contains a "pulse," assume it is an artery and do not use it. Look for another site.

- **Arterial Puncture.** Because arteries can lie close to veins, an accidental arterial puncture may occur. Arterial blood is bright red and characteristically spurts every time the heart beats. If an artery is accidentally punctured, immediately remove the catheter and control the bleeding by applying direct pressure with gauze or other dressings over the insertion site. Do not release the pressure until the hemorrhage has stopped. Typically, pressure should be held over the puncture site for a minimum of 5 minutes to stop the bleeding.

- **Circulatory Overload.** Circulatory overload occurs when an excessive amount of IV fluid is administered to a patient whose body is incapable of handling it. Common signs and symptoms of sudden circulatory overload include wet lung sounds (crackles or rales), respiratory distress, chest pain, and distention of the jugular veins . Before starting the IV, determine whether the patient has conditions or risk factors that make him or her intolerant of excessive fluid. These conditions include heart or kidney diseases or age extremes (very young or very old). Always monitor the flow rate to ensure it is appropriate for the patient's condition. If you determine that the patient is suffering from circulatory overload, slow the flow rate to TKO and sit the patient upright (if not already in an upright position). Contact medical direction for further

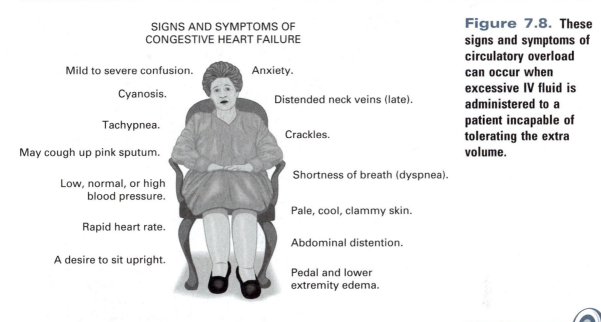

SIGNS AND SYMPTOMS OF
CONGESTIVE HEART FAILURE

Mild to severe confusion.

Cyanosis.

Tachypnea.

May cough up pink sputum.

Low, normal, or high
blood pressure.

Rapid heart rate.

A desire to sit upright.

Anxiety.

Distended neck veins (late).

Crackles.

Shortness of breath (dyspnea).

Pale, cool, clammy skin.

Abdominal distention.

Pedal and lower
extremity edema.

Figure 7.8. These signs and symptoms of circulatory overload can occur when excessive IV fluid is administered to a patient incapable of tolerating the extra volume.

treatment considerations. Figure 7.8 shows common signs and symptoms of a patient with circulatory overload.

- **Thrombophlebitis. Thrombophlebitis** describes a condition in which the vein becomes inflamed. Thrombophlebitis presents with redness and tenderness at the IV site and along the course of the vein. Generally, thrombophlebitis does not occur until several hours after the IV has been established. It is most commonly associated with long-term IV therapy. If you suspect a patient has thrombophlebitis, remove the IV and apply a warm compress to the insertion site.

- **Thrombus Formation.** A thrombus may form if the wall of the vein has been grossly injured during IV catheter insertion. As discussed previously, a thrombus may impede the movement of fluid into the patient by blocking the blood vessel or IV catheter. If a thrombus is suspected, perform the actions described in the previous section of this chapter. Do not attempt to dislodge the clot with a fluid bolus because this can cause a pulmonary embolism.

- **Air Embolism.** An **air embolism** (air bubble) is created when air enters the circulatory system through the IV catheter. Once in the circulatory system, the air bubble can travel through the veins until reaching the lungs and cause a pulmonary embolism. Air in the IV administration tubing can also enter the circulatory system and cause an air embolism. To avoid this, tamponade the distal tip of the catheter when attaching the IV tubing to the hub. Also, ensure the IV tubing has been thoroughly flushed of air and primed with IV fluid before connection to the catheter.

- **Necrosis. Necrosis** (formation and shedding of dead tissue) may occur around the catheter insertion site and is typically seen well after the IV has been placed. A primary cause of necrosis is infiltration and the extravasation of IV fluids and medications into the surrounding tissue.

On Target

Always administer IV fluid cautiously to any patient with heart failure, kidney failure, or liver disease. If a large volume of fluid must be given, continually monitor for signs of circulatory overload.

- **Anticoagulants and Hemorrhage. Anticoagulants** are medications that "thin" the blood, making it more difficult to clot. Anticoagulants are commonly used to decrease a patient's chance of suffering a stroke and/or heart attack. Medications used for anticoagulation include aspirin, Coumadin®, and heparin. When a patient is taking an anticoagulant, (such as Lovonox® or Plaux®) the chance of bleeding related to IV therapy is more likely. Control of hemorrhage is likewise more difficult, especially if an artery is inadvertently punctured. The potential for infiltration and hematoma formation is also increased. It is important to use proper technique when starting an IV on a person taking an anticoagulant and to be prepared to spend time controlling hemorrhage if it occurs.

- **Nerve and/or tendon damage.** Tendon and nerve damage can occur if you mistake a tendon or nerve for a vein and puncture either with the IV catheter. When a tendon or nerve is punctured, the patient may complain of excessive pain or the feeling of an "electrical shock" in the hand or arm. To avoid damaging a tendon or nerve, use proper technique when starting the IV and make a conscious effort to only insert the catheter where the vein lies. Avoid "blind" or haphazard attempts because this increases the chance for nerve and tendon damage.

Case Study Follow-Up

While moving a trauma patient into the ambulance, you note that the IV established prior to your arrival is not flowing properly. Immediately, you begin to scan the IV and patient for factors and conditions that may be responsible for impeding the flow of IV fluid into the patient. The IV fluid bag is at a level higher than the patient's head, and the drip chamber appears to be properly filled. Looking down toward the patient, you note that the flow regulator and slide clamps are open. Quick examination of the patient's arm indicates that the venous constricting band has been removed and there are no tight-fitting clothing that would impede the flow of IV fluid into the patient. Looking at the site where the IV has been established, you observe a hematoma accompanied by edema and redness. Recognizing infiltration, you carefully remove the IV, control the bleeding, cover the wound, and reestablish the IV in the other arm. You are successful and continue IV therapy while en route to the hospital.

■ SUMMARY

The EMT is not only accountable for establishing an IV, but also for ensuring it flows properly and any complications related to the therapy are managed appropriately. This requires the EMT to be knowledgeable and able to identify the presence of factors or conditions that will impair the flow of IV fluid into the patient, as well as complications that can arise even when an IV is properly established. Using proper technique when starting an IV and continually reassessing the status of the IV and the patient are the EMT's best defense for minimizing complications. It is also essential for the EMT to take the appropriate corrective action(s) when problems related to IV therapy are identified.

REVIEW QUESTIONS

1. You believe that the distal end of the catheter lies against a valve within the vein, therein impairing the flow of IV fluids into the patient. To correct the situation, you would
   A. remove the IV and restart it in the other extremity.
   B. carefully pull back on the IV catheter to reposition it.
   C. open the flow regulator and forcefully administer several milliliters of IV fluid.
   D. apply a warm compress over the vein.

2. For the optimal flow of IV fluid, the IV fluid bag should be positioned
   A. below the level of the IV insertion site.
   B. in front of the patient.
   C. at the level of the patient's heart.
   D. above the patient's head.

3. A thrombus has formed at the end of the catheter and is restricting the passage of IV fluid into the patient. To correct the situation, you would
   A. use a syringe filled with normal saline solution to flush the IV catheter.
   B. massage the vein to dislodge the blood clot.
   C. apply a cold compress in the area of the vein where the blood clot is located.
   D. use a syringe to aspirate the blood clot through the IV tubing.

4. Which of the following conditions would impair the flow of IV fluids into the patient?
   A. Arterial puncture
   B. Pyrogenic reaction
   C. Completely filled drip chamber
   D. Catheter shear

5. You have inserted an IV catheter into a vein and attached the administration tubing. As you open the flow regulator to administer the IV fluid to the patient, you note that the insertion site immediately becomes swollen and red. Based on this information, you would recognize
   A. localized infection.
   B. infiltration.
   C. pyrogenic reaction.
   D. circulatory overload.

6. The most common cause of a pyrogenic reaction is
   A. failure to cleanse the puncture site.
   B. patient allergy to the IV fluid.
   C. accidental puncture of a nerve.
   D. contaminated IV fluid.

7. During your annual performance review with the medical director, he asks you to describe a precaution taken to avoid causing a catheter shear when starting an IV. You would reply
   A. never pull the catheter back over the metal stylet after it has been advanced.
   B. run an IV wide open for 1 to 2 minutes to ensure all debris is removed from within the vein.
   C. never use the same vein more than once for IV therapy.
   D. massage the intended site for IV insertion prior to puncture with the IV catheter.

8. Which of the following describes the proper treatment for an accidental arterial puncture?
   A. Leave the IV catheter in place and reattempt the IV on the other extremity.
   B. Remove the IV catheter and apply a venous constricting band below the site.
   C. Remove the IV catheter and apply direct pressure with a sterile dressing until hemorrhage is controlled.
   D. Remove the IV catheter and apply a venous constricting band above the site.

9. A pyrogenic reaction typically occurs
   A. within minutes of starting IV therapy.
   B. within ½ to 1 hour of starting IV therapy.
   C. within 24 hours of starting IV therapy.
   D. within 1 week of starting IV therapy.

10. To prevent an air embolism, the EMT should
    A. tamponade the distal tip of the IV catheter when attaching the IV tubing to the catheter's hub.
    B. leave the venous constricting band in place until 100 mL of IV fluid have been administered to the patient.
    C. periodically remove the IV administration tubing from the catheter so the vein can "breathe."
    D. thoroughly cleanse the IV site with alcohol and/or betadine prior to insertion of the IV catheter.

Calculating Volumes of Fluid and IV Flow Rates

LEARNING OBJECTIVES

By the end of this section, you should be able to:

- ☑ Convert a patient's weight from pounds to kilograms
- ☑ Calculate a specific amount of IV fluid based on the patient's body weight
- ☑ Calculate a drip rate that allows a specific amount of IV fluid to be administered over a certain period of time

KEY TERMS

Drip rate—The number of drops per minute at which IV fluid must be administered so the appropriate volume of fluid can be given over a specific amount of time.

Drop factor—The number of drops required to make up 1 milliliter of IV fluid. The drop factor is always listed on the IV tubing and/or packaging.

gtt—The medical abbreviation for 1 "drop" of IV solution.

gtts—The medical abbreviation for "drops" of IV solution.

kg—The abbreviation for kilograms.

Kilograms—Metric unit of measure that describes weight.

Milliliters—Metric unit of measure that describes volume.

mL—The abbreviation for milliliters.

Case Study

You have arrived by the side of a 34-year-old male who was accidentally shot in the right upper quadrant of the abdomen with an arrow while hunting. The patient is found lying supine with the arrow protruding from his abdomen. Your assessment reveals him to be slightly confused with a patent airway and tachypneic breathing. His pulse is weak, and his skin is pale, cool, and diaphoretic. Recognizing that the patient is in shock, you and your partner apply high-flow oxygen, stabilize the arrow, and package him for rapid transport to the nearest hospital, which is 30 minutes away. Vital signs are pulse, 124 beats per minute; breathing, 28 breaths per minute; and blood pressure, 70/50 mm Hg.

While en route, you initiate an IV using a 14-gauge over-the-needle catheter and macrodrip administration tubing in the AC region of the left arm. Standing orders call for the administration of 20 milliliters per kilogram of 0.9% NSS to be delivered in sequential boluses until a systolic blood pressure of 90 mm Hg is achieved. How will you administer the IV fluid?

In Chapter 8, you learn how to calculate a specific volume of IV fluid based on a patient's weight. The calculations needed for administering a specific amount of IV fluid over a specific period of time are also presented. At the end of the chapter, we return to this case and apply your knowledge.

QUESTIONS

1. What would you do if you could not establish an IV with a 14- or 16-gauge IV catheter?
2. If the patient's systolic blood pressure was 92 mm Hg after the delivery of 900 milliliters of IV fluid, what action would you take?
3. What would happen if the EMT used the patient's weight in pounds instead of kilograms to calculate the volume of IV fluid to be administered?

■ INTRODUCTION

There may be times when administering IV fluid at a KVO/TKO or WO rate is inappropriate and perhaps harmful to the patient. Examples include pediatric patients or patients with medical conditions that make the rapid administration of IV fluids risky (e.g., heart or kidney failure). For these and other patients, medical direction may order you to administer a specific amount of IV fluid based on the patient's body weight or over a set amount of time. Performing these calculations is quite simple; however, the EMT must be proficient with basic mathematical skills such as addition, subtraction, multiplication, and division.

Calculating a Specific Volume of IV Fluid Based on the Patient's Body Weight

Administering a specific volume of IV fluid based on body weight is common when providing IV therapy to a pediatric patient or a patient in shock (especially when it comes to administering a fluid bolus). If you are to administer a specific volume of IV fluid based on the patient's weight, the medical director will typically give the order in **milliliters** or **mL** (volume) per **kilogram** or **kg** (weight). Therefore, the EMT must first convert the patient's weight from pounds to kilograms.

Converting pounds to kilograms is easy. If you have a calculator, use the following formula:

METHOD 1:

Patient weight in pounds ÷ 2.2 = Patient weight in kilograms

Examples:

- A 200-lb patient weighs **91 kg:**
  - 200 lb ÷ 2.2 = 90.9 ≈ 91 kg
- A 10-lb patient weighs **5 kg:**
  - 10 lb ÷ 2.2 = 4.5 ≈ 5 kg

Although the most accurate method of converting pounds to kilograms is by dividing the patient's weight in pounds by 2.2, a calculator may not always be available in the field. Alternative methods not involving a calculator do exist for converting pounds to kilograms, but they are not as accurate. Consequently, these methods should only be used in a "pinch."

METHOD 2:

1. Divide in half the patient's weight in pounds.
2. Determine 10% of half the patient's weight in pounds.
3. Subtract the 10% from half the patient's weight in pounds.

Examples:

- A 150-lb patient weighs **68 kg:**
  1. Half of 150 is 75
  2. 10% of 75 is 7.5
  3. 75 − 7.5 = 67.5 (rounded up is 68)
- A 300-lb patient weighs **135 kg:**
  1. Half of 300 is 150
  2. 10% of 150 is 15
  3. 150 − 15 = 135

METHOD 3:

1. Divide in half the patient's weight in pounds.
2. If the answer is in two digits, subtract the first digit. If the new figure is three digits, subtract the first two digits from it.

Examples:

- A 150-lb patient weighs **68 kg:**
  1. Half of 150 is 75
  2. 7 is the first digit
  3. 75 − 7 = 68

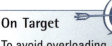
- A 300-lb patient weighs **135 kg**:
    1. Half of 300 is 150
    2. 1 and 5 are the first two digits
    3. $150 - 15 = 135$

Once the patient's body weight has been converted to kilograms, determine the total amount of IV fluid (milliliters) to be administered. This is easily accomplished using the following formula:

Milliliters (mL) × Patient weight in kilograms (kg) = Total amount of IV solution (mL)

[restated: mL × kg = total mL]

Examples:

- Medical direction has ordered 20 mL/kg of IV fluid to a 100-lb patient in shock:

    100 lb = 46 kg (100 ÷ 2.2 = 45.5)
    20 mL × 46 kg = 920 mL

    The patient would receive **920 mL** of IV fluid.

- Medical direction has ordered 20 mL/kg of IV fluid to a dehydrated 3-year-old patient weighing 40 lb:

    40 lb = 18 kg (40 ÷ 2.2 = 18.2)
    20 mL × 18 kg = 360 mL

    The patient would receive **360 mL** of IV fluid.

Administering a Specific Amount of IV Fluid Over a Specific Amount of Time

There may be times that medical direction orders you to administer a set amount of IV fluid over a specific period of time. This may be the case with pediatric patients requiring IV fluids or patients with medical conditions such as heart and/or kidney failure that make the rapid delivery of IV fluids risky to the patient's health. If required to administer a set amount of IV fluid over a specific period of time, you must calculate the appropriate flow rate.

The flow rate describes the number of drops (**gtts**) per minute that pass through the drip chamber. Calculating the flow rate is simple using the following formula:

$$\frac{\text{Volume of fluid to be administered} \times \text{Drop factor}}{\text{Time (in minutes)}} = \text{Drops (gtts) per minute}$$

- **Volume of fluid to be administered**—The volume of fluid (in milliliters) that medical direction requires to be administered.
- **Drop factor**—The **drop factor** is the number of drops required to make up 1 milliliter of IV fluid. (The drop factor is always listed on the IV tubing and/or packaging. Refer to Chapter 5 for a description and discussion of the drop factor.)

- **Time in minutes**—The period of time (in minutes) over which the IV fluid is to be administered. When using this formula, the time must always be entered as minutes. Convert hours to minutes as needed.
- **Drops per minute**—The number of drops administered over 1 minute. This is the **drip rate** and is set by adjusting the roller clamp on the IV administration tubing. **gtt** is the medical abbreviation for "drop."

Examples:

- Medical direction has ordered 300 mL of IV fluid to be given over 30 minutes to a dehydrated elderly patient with a past medical history of heart failure. The drop factor on the IV tubing is 10 gtts/mL.
  - Volume to be administered = 300 mL
  - Drop factor = 10 gtts/mL
  - Time = 30 minutes

$$\frac{300 \text{ mL} \times 10 \text{ gtts/mL}}{30 \text{ min}} = 100 \text{ drops (gtts) per minute}$$

  To administer 300 mL of IV solution over 30 minutes, you would adjust the roller clamp so **100 drops per minute** pass through the drip chamber on the IV tubing each minute. At the end of 30 minutes, 300 mL of IV fluid will have been administered.

- Medical direction has ordered 100 mL of IV fluid to be given over 2 hours to a 2-year-old patient. Microdrop administration tubing is being used with a drop factor of 60 gtts/mL.
  - Volume to be administered = 100 mL
  - Drop factor = 60 gtts/mL
  - Time = 120 minutes (2 hours)

$$\frac{100 \text{ mL} \times 60 \text{ gtts/mL}}{120 \text{ min}} = 50 \text{ drops (gtts) per minute}$$

  To administer 100 mL of IV solution over 2 hours (120 minutes), adjust the roller clamp so **50 drops per minute** passed through the drip chamber on the IV administration tubing each minute. At the end of 120 minutes (2 hours), 100 mL of IV fluid will have been administered.

> **On Target**
>
> Administering a specific volume of IV fluid (based on the patient's body weight) over a set time is an excellent way to gradually rehydrate a patient. This also avoids "overwhelming" the body with a large amount of fluid, especially if he or she has a weak heart.

Enrichment

On occasion, medical direction may order a specific amount of IV fluid based on the patient's weight to be administered over a specific amount of time—for example, when transporting a patient from one health care facility to another health care facility and a specific amount of volume is to be infused en route. This is easily calculated by performing the calculations discussed previously:

1. Convert the patient's weight in pounds to kilograms.
2. Calculate the amount of fluid to be administered based on the patient's weight in kilograms.
3. Determine the appropriate drip rate needed to administer the fluid over the predetermined amount of time.

Example:

- Medical direction has ordered 10 mL/kg of IV fluid to be administered over a 3-hour period to a dehydrated patient. The patient weighs 158 lb, and the drop factor on the IV tubing is 15 gtts/mL.

   1. 158 lb = **72 kg** (158 ÷ 2.2 = 71.8)

   2. 10 × 72 = **720 mL of IV fluid**

   3. Volume to be administered: 720 mL

   Because you are using an administration set with a drop factor of 15 gtts/mL, and you are to infuse this over 180 minutes (3 hours), you then set up the next formula:

$$\frac{720 \text{ mL } \times 15 \text{ gtts/mL}}{180 \text{ min}} = 60 \text{ drops (gtts) per minute}$$

To administer 10 mL/kg (720 mL) of IV solution over 3 hours (180 minutes), adjust the roller clamp so **60 drops per minute** (1 drop per second) pass through the drip chamber on the IV administration tubing each minute. At the end of 180 minutes (3 hours), 720 mL (10 mL/kg) of IV fluid will have been administered.

Case Study Follow-Up

You are transporting a 34-year-old male shot in the right upper quadrant of the abdomen with an arrow. The patient is in shock and exhibits the following vital signs: pulse, 124 beats per minute; breathing, 28 breaths per minute; and blood pressure, 70/50 mm Hg. You have initiated an IV in the left AC area with a 14-gauge over-the-needle catheter and macrodrip administration tubing with a drop factor of 10 gtts per milliliter. Standing orders call for the administration of 20 milliliter per kilogram of 0.9% NSS in sequential boluses until a systolic blood pressure of 90 mm Hg is achieved.

You estimate the patient to weigh 180 pounds. In your mind, you convert the patient's weight in pounds to 80 kilograms. Multiplying 20 by 80, you come up with a total volume of 1,600 milliliters of IV solution. Looking at the bag, you see that it contains 1,000 milliliters of 0.9% NSS. You open the flow regulator to allow the solution to run at a WO rate into the patient. Quickly, you establish a second IV in the left AC region using a 14-gauge IV catheter and macrodrip tubing. To give the entire 20 milliliters per kilogram bolus, you know that you will need to give 600 milliliters from the second bag once the fluid in the first bag is depleted.

As the ambulance turns into the driveway of the hospital, all fluid has been administered and the patient's systolic blood pressure is 92 mm Hg. You adjust the flow rate to a TKO/KVO setting. The patient receives a brief assessment in the emergency department and is then quickly transported to an awaiting surgical room.

■ SUMMARY

Being able to calculate a specific volume of IV fluid based on a patient's body weight or determining a drip rate that allows a specific amount of IV fluid to be administered over a specific period of time are important aspects of IV therapy. It is inappropriate to believe that all infusion rates are either TKO/KVO or WO. Although TKO/KVO is the most common flow rate and WO is usually reserved for the hypovolemic trauma victim, a mind-set that "all" patients should receive fluid at a KVO or WO rate cannot be assumed. Simply apply and use the formulas presented in this section to easily calculate specific volumes of IV fluid based on body weight and appropriate drip rates necessary to administer a set amount of IV fluid over a specified amount of time.

REVIEW QUESTIONS

1. Covert the following weights in pounds to kilograms using all three conversion methods:

	Method 1	Method 2	Method 3
a. 120 lb	____ kg	____ kg	____ kg
b. 40 lb	____ kg	____ kg	____ kg
c. 400 lb	____ kg	____ kg	____ kg
d. 10 lb	____ kg	____ kg	____ kg
e. 80 lb	____ kg	____ kg	____ kg
f. 250 lb	____ kg	____ kg	____ kg

2. Medical command orders a 20 mL/kg bolus to a dehydrated 65-year-old male patient. The patient weighs 140 lb. How much IV fluid will you administer?

   A. 2,800 mL
   B. 128 mL
   C. 640 mL
   D. 1,280 mL
   E. None of the above

3. Medical command orders a 10 mL/kg bolus to a 2-year-old patient requiring IV therapy. The patient weighs 16 lb. How much IV fluid will you administer?

   A. 70 mL
   B. 140 mL
   C. 160 mL
   D. 260 mL
   E. None of the above

4. You must administer 500 mL of IV fluid using IV administration tubing with a drop factor of 15 gtts/mL. How many drops per minute are required to administer this volume over 60 minutes?

    A. 18 gtts/min

    B. 125 gtts/min

    C. 2,000 gtts/min

    D. 80 gtts/min

    E. None of the above

5. You must administer 250 mL using IV administration tubing with a drop factor of 60 gtts/mL. How many drops per minute are required to administer this volume over 3 hours?

    A. 48 gtts/min

    B. 62 gtts/min

    C. 78 gtts/min

    D. 83 gtts/min

    E. None of the above

Special Patient Considerations

LEARNING OBJECTIVES

By the end of this chapter, you should be able to:

- ☑ Identify special considerations of IV therapy when managing a pediatric patient
- ☑ Identify special considerations of IV therapy when managing a geriatric patient
- ☑ Identify special considerations of IV therapy when managing an obese patient
- ☑ Identify special considerations of IV therapy when managing a patient with a medical condition intolerant of excess fluid
- ☑ Identify special considerations of IV therapy when managing a multisystems trauma patient or patient with a serious medical condition

KEY TERMS

Contractures—Flexion of a joint, typically permanent. Contractures typically occur during the slow degeneration of the musculoskeletal system found with many chronic disease states.

Crackles—Moist breath sounds indicating the accumulation of fluid in the lung tissue. Crackles are also referred to as "rales."

Geriatric—Person older than 65 years of age.

Golden hour—Trauma care guideline stating that a patient's best chance for surviving serious injury(s) occurs when surgical intervention is provided within 1 hour of injury.

Pediatric—An infant or child. Generally accepted as any patient younger than 18 years of age, although criteria for specific age brackets do exist.

Platinum 10 minutes—Trauma care guideline stating that EMS should spend no longer than 10 minutes at the scene with a traumatically injured patient (barring access issues such as entrapment).

Case Study

You are called to respond to a 2-year-old male with an unknown medical problem. At the scene, you find the child actively seizing. A paramedic unit has also been dispatched but is 20 minutes away. The mother informs you that her son does not have a history of seizures and has not been sick or had a fever. Since your patient's condition is poor, you provide high-flow oxygen, and then move him onto the stretcher and into the ambulance for transport. His panic-stricken mother gets into the front seat of the ambulance. Three minutes into the transport, the patient stops seizing.

Knowing that paramedics will administer an antiseizure medication if the child seizes again, you prepare to start an IV while he is not seizing. How will you alter your approach and technique to start the IV on the child?

In Chapter 9, you learn about special patients and conditions that may force you to alter your approach and technique when providing IV therapy. Specific tips relating to specific patients and conditions are also discussed. At the end of the chapter, we return to this case and apply your knowledge.

QUESTIONS

1. Given that the patient is not hypovolemic, at what rate would you administer the IV fluid and what would you specifically assess to determine whether the patient is becoming overloaded with IV fluid?

2. Would it be equally acceptable to not start the IV, given that the patient is no longer seizing?

3. Why is it a good idea to keep the mother informed of what is happening, not only when starting the IV, but regarding overall care?

■ INTRODUCTION

There will be times when you are faced with special patients or circumstances that present challenges to starting and/or maintaining an IV. Examples include patients that are young, old, obese, or have medical conditions that make them intolerant of excess fluid. Situations such as major trauma or other medical conditions may also force you to tailor your care involving IV therapy. This section provides you with basic information for these special patients so the most effective IV therapy and patient care can be provided.

Pediatrics

Starting an IV on a sick or injured **pediatric** patient can be extremely challenging, not to mention stressful. A child's ability to fully understand a medical emergency and the necessary treatment is often limited. Fear and panic are common reactions that typically result in crying, screaming, and failure to remain still for placement of an IV. Because children tend to be less tolerant of pain, insertion of the sharp venipuncture device contributes to behaviors that make placing an IV difficult. Compounding this is the fact that you are a stranger to the child. When starting an IV on a pediatric, consider the following:

- **Anatomical and Physiological Considerations**
  - Pediatrics are different than adults in regard to their anatomical and physiological makeup. Infant's and children's veins are smaller, making IV placement more challenging. Because the amount of fat tends to be increased on infants and young children, finding already small veins is more difficult. Once the IV has been placed, spasms of the vein can impair the flow of fluid into the infant's or child's body.
  - Because the immune system of an infant or young child is not as developed as that of a healthy adult, any infection secondary to IV therapy can be devastating. Therefore, it is critical to thoroughly cleanse the skin of microorganisms prior to catheter insertion and to cover the site after the IV has been established.
  - The developing heart and kidneys in an infant or child make him or her less tolerant of fluid overload. Careful monitoring of the flow rate and use of microdrip or volume-controlled administration tubing is encouraged, unless the patient requires the rapid administration of fluid or blood. Constant assessment for the signs and symptoms of fluid overload is critical. See the Excess Fluid Intolerance section later in this chapter for further discussion.
- **Gaining IV Access in Pediatrics.** Because gaining IV access in pediatrics can be difficult, consider the following tips:
  - **Have Adequate Help.** When starting an IV on an infant or child, always make sure you have adequate help. Use parents or caregivers when appropriate to provide emotional and physical support to the infant or child.
  - **Position the Patient.** The exact position of the EMT and the patient will be determined by what vessel will be used. It is best to position yourself at the same level as the patient if possible, in a position that enables you to clearly see and cannulate the vein. Because starting IVs on children is often difficult, do everything you can to make your first attempt successful.
  - **Explain the Procedure.** If the child is old enough to understand, explain why you are starting the IV and describe each step as you do it in terms he or she can understand. This may help prepare him or her and avoid surprises that can result in panic, crying, and screaming, or other noncompliant behavior. Never tell the patient

On Target

Never tell a pediatric patient or the parents or caregivers that the IV will not hurt. IVs do hurt when being inserted, and all involved must be prepared for this. Failure to be honest can create an environment of distrust and poor compliance with IV placement or additional care.

On Target

Remember that family members or caregivers are considered patients when dealing with a pediatric. Therefore, if possible, inform them of what is happening and use them to help calm a panic-stricken child. This can go a long way in successfully placing an IV and in providing any additional care.

that the IV will not hurt. Rather, tell the patient that he or she will feel some pain, but it will be over very quickly. Also, do not reveal the needle or talk too much about the discomfort associated with IV therapy too early, this may result in increasing the child's anxiety and bring about noncompliant behavior. Be confident and keep the parent(s) or other caregivers informed of what is occurring. Cooperative and supportive parents go a long way toward getting a child to comply with your needs.

On Target

Because IVs in scalp veins are time consuming and difficult to place, they are rarely used in the prehospital setting. It is easiest and best to place an IV in the extremity of a pediatric. Never use the scalp for IV access unless the patient is in critical condition and all other attempts have proven unsuccessful (assuming medical direction allows EMTs to use the scalp for IV therapy).

- **Site Selection.** When attempting IV access in pediatrics, always look to the upper extremities for initial access. Scalp veins are sometimes considered for newborns and young infants in an emergent situation (in the absence of an identifiable extremity site), but it is more time consuming and complicated. Hair must often be removed, and stabilization of the IV is difficult due to the curvature of the skull. In addition, arteries in the scalp lie closer to the surface of the skin than in the extremities, making an inadvertent arterial puncture more likely. Never use scalp veins for IV therapy unless local medical direction permits.

- **Consider a Warm Compress.** When looking for a suitable vein, consider applying a warm compress to the site while using a venous constricting band. The warm compress may help distend veins, making them more visible and easier to access.

- **Consider Smaller IV Catheters.** Twenty-two- and 24-gauge IV catheters are frequently required due to the smaller size of pediatric blood vessels. Also, consider inserting the venipuncture device with the bevel down, as opposed to in an up position. This enables the return of blood as soon as the stylet enters the vein, decreasing the chance of the catheter continuing through the other side of the vessel wall, resulting in infiltration.

On Target

It is extremely discouraging, and detrimental to patient care, to successfully place an IV in a pediatric, only to have it dislodged by the patient or by patient movement. Therefore, once the IV has been placed, take extra care to make sure it is secured appropriately.

- **Securing the IV.** Once the IV has been established, securing it becomes a priority. A moving or curious child may inadvertently dislodge the IV, which necessitates reattempting the IV. Consider gently wrapping the IV tubing to the arm with roller gauze. However, make sure to leave the insertion site and any medication administration ports uncovered so you can monitor for complications and allow the delivery of IV medications. Do not apply the roller gauze so tightly that it compresses the arm and limits the flow of IV fluid into the patient. Immobilization or soft restraint of the extremity may be required to prevent movement and dislodgment of the IV (Figure 9.1). If in doubt, follow local medical direction.

For a critical pediatric patient, it may be best to establish the IV en route because successful placement of an IV is often difficult and may waste valuable time by delaying transport. Some EMS systems limit the number of IV attempts on an infant or child, necessitating the contact of medical direction if an IV cannot be established after the first or second attempt. If ALS providers are at the scene or are meeting with you en route,

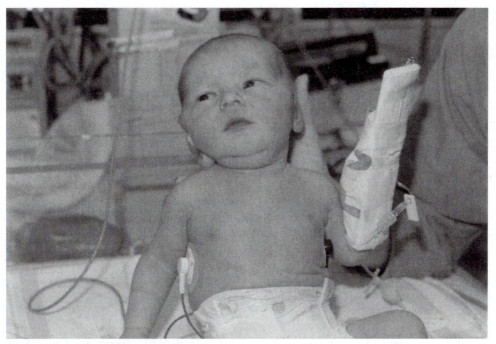

Figure 9.1. The use of an arm splint in very young patients will help avoid accidental dislodgment of the IV line.

they may obtain venous access by using intraosseous cannulation (inserting a needle into a bone) in the critical patient. In any instance, follow local medical direction.

Geriatrics

A large number of EMS responses involve **geriatrics,** or persons older than 65 years of age. Like children, geriatrics can present challenges to IV therapy for various reasons. Consider the following when starting an IV on a geriatric patient:

- **Anatomical and Physiological Considerations**
  - With age, veins become thicker, less elastic, and hardened. This makes establishing the IV, as well as the delivery of IV fluids into the circulatory system, more difficult. The flash of blood seen in the flashback chamber of the venipuncture device may not be as pronounced as in younger, healthier patients, making it more difficult to determine whether the catheter is in a vein. Veins become less anchored as the adipose in the subcutaneous layer of the skin diminishes, allowing them to "roll" when inserting the IV catheter. Valves are more prominent and are often hardened by calcium and plaque. This makes threading the catheter into the vein difficult. Some elderly patients also have what are called "spider veins," which are very small blood vessels near the surface of the skin.

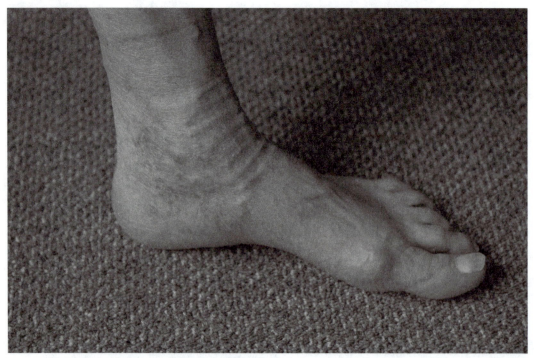

Figure 9.2. **Spider veins are small, peripheral dilated veins that are easy to locate, but essentially impossible to cannulate. These vessels should always be avoided.**

Over time, spider veins become engorged due to excessive back pressure in the venous system. These veins, although easy to see, are not to be used for IV therapy (Figure 9.2).

On Target

For geriatrics with delicate skin, special paper tape is often preferred over conventional medical tape, which is stickier and increases the risk of a skin tear when the IV is removed or must be changed.

- Body organs and systems decline with age. The skin of older patients can be thin and fragile, and is prone to injury during puncture with an IV angiocatheter. The skin may also tear from tape used to secure the administration tubing to the patient's arm and from the protective membrane placed over the site of insertion. Careful taping is paramount.

- Decline of the immune system leaves the elderly patient prone to infection. Once an infection originates, it can spread throughout the body and be extremely difficult to treat. Therefore, it is critical that the site be thoroughly cleansed with alcohol and/or betadine prior to attempting the IV.

- Declining heart and/or kidney function leave the patient prone to complications from excessive fluid administration or fluid overload. See the Excess Fluid Intolerance section later in this chapter for more discussion on how to avoid fluid overload on a fluid-intolerant geriatric.

- **Medical Conditions**
    - Cognitive diseases or conditions that affect the brain (e.g., Alzheimer's, dementia, stroke) are more prevalent in the later years of life. Patients with these conditions may not appreciate that you are

there to help them, not hurt them. This can lead to thrashing and combativeness, making IV placement and ongoing therapy challenging.

- Debilitated patients may also have **contractures** (flexion of a joint, typically permanent) of the hands and arms, making finding a suitable site for IV therapy a formidable task.

- Preexisting medical conditions must always be considered when performing IV therapy on the geriatric patient. Medical conditions such as heart or renal disease can impair the person's ability to process or tolerate excess body fluid. Continually monitor fluid administration and consider smaller-gauge IVs, as well as microdrip or volume-controlled administration tubing, for geriatric patients that do not require large amounts of fluid.

- Diseases such as cancer and the use of steroids can also decrease immune function, leaving geriatric patients more susceptible to infection. Ensure an IV site has been adequately cleaned with alcohol and/or betadine prior to catheter insertion.

- A significant portion of elderly patients also take medications that "thin" their blood (e.g., Coumadin, aspirin, heparin). These medications may make the control of hemorrhage more difficult and may result in significant bruising or the formation of hematomas secondary to unsuccessful catheterization of the vein.

- **Gaining IV Access in Geriatrics.** Because performing IV therapy on a geriatric patient can be difficult, along with the normal considerations given to any patients in need of IV therapy, these additional tips may be beneficial:

  - **Site Selection.** Feel and select "spongy" veins, not veins that are hard. The walls of hard veins contain calcium and plaque, making them harder to access and slide the IV catheter into. Fluid delivery through such veins is often less than optimal. Avoid areas in which the catheter will pass through or otherwise contact a valve. Valves can interfere with the placement of the catheter and block the delivery of IV fluid. Because the veins may be less well anchored by a diminished subcutaneous layer, manually stabilize the veins with your nondominant hand when placing the catheter. Along with the tendency of veins to "roll" due to a lack of subcutaneous tissue, they can also become more torturous. Figure 9.3 shows an adult forearm alongside a geriatric forearm. Note the difference in the appearance of the skin and veins, and how the veins course up the arm.

  - **Venous Constricting Band.** Never leave the venous constricting band in place for too long (greater than 2 minutes) or apply too tightly. Leaving the band in place for too long can injure the skin and blood vessels, as well as rupture a delicate vein by creating significant back pressure. Applying the band too tightly may also result in localized bruising and injury, especially if the patient is on blood thinners. One way to alleviate this concern is to use a blood

On Target

If an IV attempt is unsuccessful and the patient is taking an anticoagulant, be prepared to control the associated bleeding. A pressure dressing may be required.

On Target

For the geriatric with delicate skin and fragile blood vessels, a blood pressure cuff instead of the venous constricting band may be preferable to occlude venous blood flow and dilate the veins. Pressure applied by the blood pressure cuff is distributed over a greater surface and is more subtle than the pressure associated with the venous constricting band. When using a blood pressure cuff, inflate it to 20 mm Hg less than the patient's systolic blood pressure.

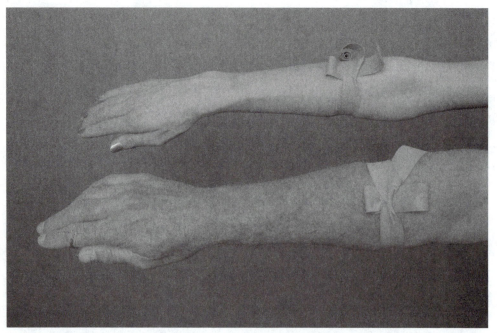

Figure 9.3. Photo comparing the skin appearance, forearm structure, and vein prominence in a young adult versus a geriatric patient. Veins commonly become harder to find as a person ages.

pressure cuff instead of an elastic constricting band. Just be sure to only inflate the cuff enough to impede venous flow. This is best accomplished by inflating the cuff 20 mm Hg less than the patient's systolic pressure.

- **Proper IV Supplies and Materials.** Carefully select the proper IV supplies and materials. Smaller-gauge catheters may be required. Never use a catheter larger than what the vein will handle. The use of microdrip IV tubing or a volume-controlled administration set may be advantageous to limit the amount of fluid the patient receives, unless significant volume is immediately required.

Obesity

Obese patients present challenges when performing IV therapy because the increased deposition of fat makes locating veins much more difficult. If a vein is not readily visible, carefully palpate potential sites for underlying veins. Never attempt to place an IV catheter in a blood vessel that pulsates because it is most likely an artery. It is extremely helpful to have an appreciation of the typical layout of veins in the hands, arms, and AC. This will help you find veins by palpating in areas where veins "should be." Once a potential vein is located, place the IV as you would with any other patient. Figure 9.4 shows how obesity can obscure veins and subsequently impact site selection.

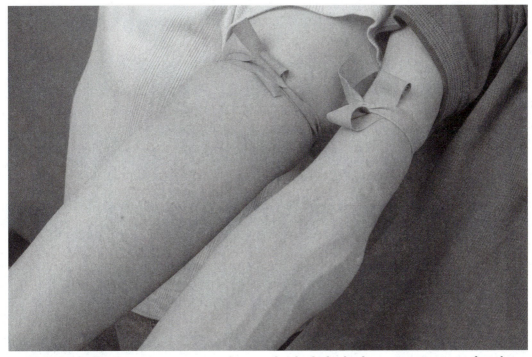

Figure 9.4. Notice how the presence of excessive body fat in these two same-age females effectively "hides" the peripheral veins.

Fluid Intolerance

Patients with heart conditions, liver disease, and/or kidney failure may be less tolerant of excess fluid than otherwise healthy individuals. Infants and very young children also cannot tolerate excessive fluid due to developing body systems. Actively assess for such conditions by relating a patient's age to body system development or decline, along with asking the patient or caregiver about medical conditions that can put him or her at a disadvantage for handling extra fluid in the body. (See Chapter 7 for more on fluid overload.)

If the patient is intolerant of excess fluid, adjust the flow rate accordingly. Some EMS systems may opt for placement of a heparin or saline lock, instead of administration tubing and IV fluid. (Heparin or saline locks are discussed in Chapter 10.) Use of a microdrip administration set or measured volume administration set may be indicated, unless the rapid infusion of volume is necessary.

Continually monitor the patient for signs and symptoms of fluid overload. Patients with excess body fluid typically complain of shortness of breath and possibly chest pain. At a minimum, auscultate breath sounds every few minutes and use a pulse oximeter if available. The presence of moist breath sounds like **"crackles"** and/or a declining pulse-oximetry reading indicate possible fluid overload. If the patient begins to experience fluid overload, sit the patient upright (if not contraindicated) and slow the IV to a KVO rate. Follow local protocol or contact medical direction for additional actions.

On Target

For the patient with medical conditions intolerant of excess IV fluid, constantly monitor the flow rate and continually assess for signs of fluid overload. If the patient becomes overloaded, sit him or her upright and contact medical direction for further treatment.

Trauma Patients

The role of IV therapy when caring for a severely injured trauma patient is controversial. A critically injured patient in shock requires timely surgical care to definitively repair his or her injuries. Prehospital care is limited to essential stabilization and primarily revolves around airway management, hemorrhage control, and rapid transport to the most appropriate hospital. The concept of the **"golden hour"** reveals that the best opportunity for recovery occurs if the patient receives surgical intervention within 1 hour of his or her injury.

The **"platinum 10 minutes"** conveys the concept that EMS personnel should spend no longer than 10 minutes on scene with a trauma patient (unless entrapment or patient access is an issue), performing only the most essential treatments (e.g., airway, hemorrhage control, and immobilization).

When managing a critically injured trauma patient, emergency physicians and trauma surgeons affirm that IV placement and therapy should be attempted while en route to the hospital. Attempting IV access at the scene wastes valuable time and will delay the patient's access to the surgical suite (unless you function within a first-responder system that does not provide transport or are waiting for an aeromedical helicopter).

The best replacement for lost blood is blood. IV crystalloids and colloids do not carry oxygen; thus, the administration of blood will allow additional oxygen to be delivered to the cells. Although blood does carry oxygen to the cells, few if any field services carry it due to scant supply and specific storage requirements. Blood substitutes do provide promise but remain experimental at the present time.

The EMT, however, can alter his or her approach to setting up the IV in the trauma victim, which then allows easier administration of blood once at the hospital. The EMT should use a blood administration set if the patient is a victim of trauma and is likely to receive blood at the hospital. If it turns out that the patient does not need blood at the hospital, you will still have a patent IV line for crystalloid and medication administration. If the patient is in need of blood, having blood tubing already in place will save valuable time at the hospital because there will not be a need to change out the administration set.

The role of volume replacement and blood pressure in the trauma patient is controversial. Often, emergency physicians and surgeons prefer to maintain a lower blood pressure rather than a higher blood pressure. A systolic blood pressure between 80 and 100 mm Hg is adequate to perfuse the cells of the body's most critical organs (heart, brain, lungs, and kidneys), but not high enough to destroy blood clots forming within the body in areas where the blood vessels have been damaged and bleeding is occurring.

The amount of IV crystalloid to administer to the trauma patient is frequently dependent on the patient's weight. Typically, 20 milliliter per kilogram is suggested for the adult or young child, whereas 10 milliliter per kilogram is used for an infant younger than 30 days. After calculating the appropriate volume, the fluid is generally administered at a WO rate until the desired volume has been delivered or the patient's systolic blood pressure is at an acceptable level (see Chapter 8 for calculating volumes of IV fluid

On Target

For the critical trauma patient, always start the IV en route, unless the patient is entrapped and IV access can be established. Definitive care for the traumatized patient lies in the surgical suite and must be performed as quickly as possible. Delaying transport at the scene to start an IV wastes valuable time and may contribute to a less than favorable patient outcome.

On Target

Always use macrodrip or blood tubing for the traumatized patient.

based on the patient's weight). Follow medical direction concerning IV therapy and the acceptable blood pressure to attain in the trauma patient.

Patients with Critical Medical Conditions

For patients suffering from severe medical conditions such as stroke, cardiac compromise, shock, or heart failure, definitive care is only available in the hospital. Often, the effectiveness of the definitive care is time dependent and must be administered as quickly as possible. IV therapy at the scene may delay access to the necessary critical care and contribute to a less than desirable outcome. Therefore, many medical directors and emergency physicians recommend providing IV therapy while en route to the hospital as opposed to at the scene. Follow local medical direction concerning IV therapy and the patient with a critical medical condition.

Case Study Follow-Up

You must initiate an IV on a 2-year-old pediatric who was in active seizures on your arrival. The seizure activity has since subsided, but an IV is required in the event that the patient reseizes. Paramedics will meet you en route to the hospital; if the IV is already established, they can immediately administer an anticonvulsant medication. To complicate an already stressful situation, the boy's panic-stricken mother is in the front seat of the ambulance.

Quickly, you mentally review some of the basic differences between pediatric and adult patients, including the smaller veins found in the child and the fact that young children tend to be less tolerant of excessive fluid due to a maturing heart and kidneys. After inspecting potential IV sites, you select a 22-gauge venipuncture device and microdrip administration tubing. You prepare the IV tubing and bag of IV fluid as you would for an adult patient.

Noticing that the patient's mother is watching from the front seat, you take the time to explain why you are starting the IV and describe each step as you perform it. You successfully place the IV in the patient's left arm and then secure the IV tubing with roller gauze since the patient is slightly combative and there is a risk of dislodgment. The mother seems somewhat more at ease with your proficiency and knowledge.

Paramedics rendezvous at the meeting site and climb on board. Approximately 5 minutes later, the patient seizes again. Because an IV is already in place, the paramedic administers an anticonvulsant medication, which promptly stops the seizure activity.

At the hospital, it is determined that the young boy ingested some of his grandmother's medication, causing him to seize. He is treated in the emergency department and then transferred to the pediatric intensive care unit where he spends 1 week before being released home. No permanent brain or organ damage was noted.

■ SUMMARY

There will be times when special patients or circumstances will force you to modify your approach to IV therapy. Examples include patients who are very young or old, as well as conditions such as obesity, trauma, and pre-existing medical problems that are intolerant of excessive fluid administration. It is the responsibility of the EMT to have a basic understanding of these patients and conditions, and of the appropriate modifications to be taken. Doing so will not only enable optimal IV therapy, but will also allow the EMT to provide the best patient care possible.

REVIEW QUESTIONS

1. Starting an IV on a pediatric may be more difficult than on an adult because
   A. the amount of fat is decreased on a young child compared with a healthy adult.
   B. veins are not yet formed in the young pediatric.
   C. children tend to have spider veins.
   D. the veins of a pediatric tend to be smaller than an adult's veins.

2. The developing heart and kidneys of an infant or child make him or her less tolerant of fluid overload than a healthy adult.
   A. True
   B. False

3. Which of the following statements is most appropriate to tell a young child when starting an IV on him or her?
   A. "This will not hurt at all."
   B. "Act like a grown-up and deal with the pain."
   C. "The more you fuss, the more it will hurt."
   D. "You may feel some pain, but it will be over quickly."

4. Which of the following IV catheters would most likely be the easiest to place in a pediatric patient?
   A. 14 Gauge
   B. 16 Gauge
   C. 18 Gauge
   D. 22 Gauge

5. You have started an IV on a 3-year-old patient and secured it using roller gauze. When applying the roller gauze, you must ensure
   A. macrodrip tubing has been used.
   B. the medication ports are left uncovered.
   C. the gauze is applied tightly enough to block venous but not arterial blood flow.
   D. the insertion site is covered with gauze to prevent contamination.

6. When placing an IV in a geriatric patient, the EMT must remember that
   A. veins tend to be thicker, hardened, and less elastic.
   B. spider veins present good opportunities for IV access.
   C. veins are well anchored by increased amounts of adipose tissue.
   D. skin thickens, making IV access more challenging.

7. You are starting an IV on a geriatric patient who takes aspirin. This is important to the EMT because
   A. the patient will feel less pain when the IV is placed.
   B. there is no need to clean the skin with alcohol prior to starting the IV.
   C. alcohol should be avoided and betadine used to clean the patient's skin prior to puncture.
   D. there is greater chance that bleeding associated with the IV may occur.

8. Which of the following tips is helpful when starting an IV in an obese patient?
   A. "Blind" sticks must be used in an attempt to locate a vein.
   B. The angle of inserting a venipuncture device must be increased to between 45 and 90 degrees.
   C. Placement of the IV in an artery is permissible if a vein cannot be located and the patient is in critical condition.
   D. Having an appreciation of the typical layout of blood vessels is advantageous.

9. You are providing IV therapy to a patient with renal failure, predisposing him to complications from fluid overload. Which of the following signs would indicate that the patient has received too much fluid?
   A. Hypotension
   B. Shortness of breath
   C. Low blood sugar
   D. Back pain

10. As a general rule, which of the following statements is true concerning IV access and the critical trauma patient.
    A. IV access should be initiated prior to transport so lifesaving fluids can be administered.
    B. IV access should be attempted while en route to the hospital.
    C. IV therapy should incorporate microdrip tubing.
    D. IV access should be avoided.

11. For the trauma patient, which of the following is true related to prehospital IV therapy?
    A. The best replacement for lost blood is normal saline solution.
    B. Blood tubing should be used when possible.

    C. Blood can be easily administered by EMTs in the field setting, given approval by medical direction.

    D. IV crystalloids are extremely beneficial because they can carry oxygen to the cells.

12. While infusing a 2,000-milliliter bolus of 0.9% normal saline to a patient, he starts to complain of dyspnea. You note the pulse oximeter reading is dropping and auscultate crackles in the bases of the lungs. Based on this information, you would realize

    A. an improper IV solution has been administered.

    B. the patient is about to have a seizure.

    C. the patient is becoming overloaded with fluid.

    D. the flow rate of the IV solution must be increased.

13. What would your immediate action be in caring for the patient in question 12?

    A. Change to another IV solution.

    B. Prepare to care for a seizure patient.

    C. Stop the fluid bolus and set the flow rate at KVO.

    D. Increase the flow rate.

14. You are managing a trauma patient and have established two large-bore IVs. After a fluid bolus of 2,000 milliliters, the patient exhibits a systolic blood pressure of 92 mm Hg. At this point, you would

    A. contact medical control for permission to repeat the fluid bolus.

    B. repeat the fluid bolus without contacting medical control.

    C. slow one IV to KVO and keep the other running WO.

    D. slow both IVs to KVO and contact medical direction.

15. You are administering IV fluids to a patient during an interfacility transport. Halfway through the trip, you note that the patient is showing signs of fluid overload. You should

    A. keep the fluid running as directed and contact medical direction.

    B. slow the IV to KVO and contact medical direction.

    C. keep the fluid running as directed until the paramedic rendezvous with your squad.

    D. shut down the IV and disconnect it from the patient.

Special Procedures

LEARNING OBJECTIVES

By the end of this chapter, you should be able to:

☑ Describe the procedure for removing a peripheral IV

☑ Describe the procedure for changing IV administration tubing

☑ Differentiate a saline lock from a standard IV and explain indications for its use

☑ Describe the procedure for placing a saline lock

☑ List the equipment needed to draw venous blood from an IV catheter

☑ Describe the procedure of obtaining venous blood from an IV catheter with a blood tube holder, luer lock, and blood tubes, as well as a 20-milliliter syringe

KEY TERMS

Blood tube holder—A device into which blood tubes are inserted when obtaining venous blood from an IV catheter.

Blood tubes—Glass or plastic tubes used to obtain and store venous blood.

Luer lock—Special adapter that fits into the blood tube holder and permits blood to be transferred from the IV catheter into the blood tube.

Saline lock—A device used for IV access that does not incorporate IV administration tubing or a bag of IV fluid.

Vacutainer—See Blood tube holder.

Venous blood sampling—The process by which venous blood is withdrawn from the IV catheter and placed in blood tubes for laboratory analysis.

Case Study

You work in a rural county and are transporting a 46-year-old female to another medical facility approximately 2 hours away after she came to the hospital with a large laceration to the right hand from a table saw. Because the laceration involved damage to the tendons and nerves, the patient is being transferred to a surgeon who specializes in hand injuries. Prior to transport, all hemorrhage was controlled and an IV of 0.9% NSS was initiated in the left forearm with a 16-gauge catheter. The IV has been running at a rate between TKO and WO.

During transport, you realize that the IV fluid bag is almost empty. Because it will be another 45 minutes before you arrive at the receiving facility, you must hang a new bag of IV fluid. How will you accomplish this?

In Chapter 10, you will learn about procedures related to IV therapy beyond initiating an IV. As an EMT permitted to initiate IV lines, it will also be expected that you know how to perform other common skills associated with the procedure. These skills often include (but are not limited to), IV removal, drawing blood, and changing the IV solution bag or administration set due to medical direction or a need dictated by the patient's condition. At the end of the chapter, we return to this case and apply your knowledge.

QUESTIONS

1. What action(s) would you take if, while changing the IV fluid bag the exposed spike of the IV tubing fell onto the ground?
2. Why is it advantageous to use the slide clamp to stop the flow of IV fluid when changing the IV fluid bag?
3. Is it necessary to change the primary IV tubing any time the IV fluid bag needs to be replaced?

■ INTRODUCTION

The EMT may have to perform other activities related to IV therapy aside from its initiation and maintenance. Medical direction may order the EMT to change fluids or IV tubing after the IV has been placed and running. An IV may have to be removed if it has infiltrated or is otherwise nonpatent. Some EMS systems may also require EMTs to obtain venous blood samples while starting an IV or inserting a saline lock.

Removing a Peripheral IV

An IV that is infiltrated or will not flow (after considering any and all problems) must be removed. Use the following procedure to remove an IV:

1. Take appropriate BSI precautions.

2. Stop the flow of IV fluid through the administration tubing by moving the slide clamps or flow regulator to a closed position.

3. Remove all tape or other securing materials from the IV tubing and catheter. When possible, remove adhesive material in the same direction as the hair pattern on the arm to minimize the discomfort.

4. Place a sterile gauze pad over the area where the IV catheter has been inserted into the skin and apply gentle pressure with the fingers or thumb of your nondominant hand.

5. Grasp the catheter by the hub and swiftly remove it by pulling straight back. Be careful how you handle the catheter because blood splattering may occur.

6. Apply direct pressure with the sterile gauze until the bleeding has stopped.

7. Cover the site with an adhesive bandage or clean gauze and tape to protect against infection.

8. Periodically recheck the site for spontaneous bleeding and provide corrective treatment as needed.

Drain any IV fluid remaining in bag. Dispose of the empty bag, IV tubing, and catheter, as well as the gauze used to control any bleeding, in a biohazard bag. If a butterfly catheter was used, dispose of the catheter in a needle disposal container.

On Target

Just as when an IV is inserted, it is critical that the EMT is careful not to contaminate the site after the IV has been removed. This involves not touching the insertion site and covering it with a sterile dressing. Some systems advocate applying an antibiotic gel to the insertion site prior to covering.

Changing IV Administration Tubing

There may be times when the IV administration tubing must be changed after the IV has been established. To change the IV administration tubing, use the following procedure:

1. Take appropriate BSI precautions.

2. Prepare a new IV fluid bag with the new IV tubing as described in Chapter 6.

3. Stop the flow of IV fluid through the administration tubing by moving the slide clamps or flow regulator to a closed position.

4. Remove the tape securing the IV tubing to the patient's arm.

5. Gently press downward over top of the vein where the tip of the catheter or metal stylet (butterfly catheter) lies to prevent blood from flowing back through the catheter and air from entering the circulatory system.

6. Carefully detach the IV tubing from the hub of the catheter.

7. Insert the needle adapter of the new IV tubing into the catheter's hub.

8. Open the slide clamp and/or regulator.

9. Administer several milliliters of IV fluid to ensure patency.

10. Set the proper flow rate using the flow regulator.

11. Tape the new IV administration tubing to the patient's arm.

Dispose of the old IV tubing in a biohazard container. Like any other aspect of IV therapy, changing the IV administration tubing is a sterile

On Target

The use of extension tubing, or the small tubing used to start a saline lock (discussed later), makes changing IV tubing much easier. When extension tubing or the tubing of a saline lock is in place, the EMT does not have to remove the primary IV tubing from the IV catheter (only remove it from the end of the extension tubing or saline lock tubing), decreasing the risk of dislodgment and infection.

process. If at any time the new bag, IV tubing, or catheter becomes contaminated, dispose of these items and restart with new materials.

Changing an IV Fluid Bag

If medical direction orders a different IV fluid for administration or the IV bag is nearly empty (less than 50 milliliters of fluid), you will have to change the IV fluid bag. To change the IV fluid bag, use the following procedure:

1. Take appropriate BSI precautions.
2. Remove the protective cover over the administration set port on the new bag of IV fluid.
3. Stop the flow of IV fluid into the IV tubing using the slide clamp, not the flow control (this eliminates the need to recalibrate the flow rate).
4. Remove the IV tubing from the depleted IV bag.
5. Insert the spike into the new IV bag.
6. Squeeze the drip chamber if necessary to ensure it is filled with the appropriate amount of IV fluid.
7. Move the slide clamp into the open position and reverify the drip rate is as desired.

On Target

Using the slide clamp to stop the flow of IV fluid from the bag into the patient is better than using the flow regulator because the EMT will not have to reset the flow rate.

If a noticeable amount of air becomes entrained within the IV tubing while changing the IV bag, cleanse a medication administration port below the trapped air and insert with a hypodermic needle attached if the tubing is not needleless (attach only the syringe if using a needleless system). Pull back on the plunger to move the trapped air from the tubing and into the syringe.

Remember that changing an IV bag is a sterile process. If at any time the new bag or existing IV tubing becomes contaminated, dispose of the contaminated items and start again with new materials. Drain any remaining IV fluid from the old bag and dispose of it in a biohazard bag.

Enrichment

Saline Lock

Saline locks (once called heparin locks because heparin was periodically injected to keep blood clots from forming at the end of the IV catheter) are similar to traditional IVs, but do not use IV tubing or a bag of IV fluid. Saline locks are used by many EMS systems for patients not requiring fluid or for whom the IV is being placed for precautionary reasons only. Like a traditional IV, a saline lock uses a catheter placed directly into a vein. However, instead of IV administration tubing, it uses very short tubing with a clamp and a distal medication port.

Placing a saline lock requires the following materials (Figure 10.1):

- Venipuncture device
- Saline lock

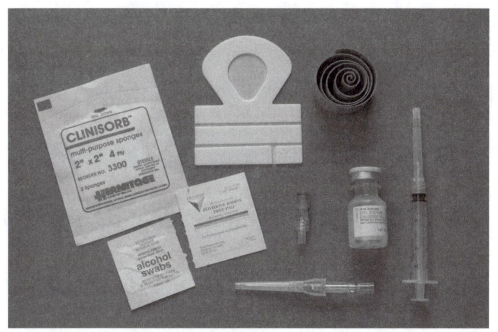

Figure 10.1. Common equipment needed to initiate vascular access using a saline lock.

- Syringe with 3 cc to 5 cc of sterile saline
- Tape or commercial securing device
- Venous blood-drawing equipment (as needed)
- Venous constricting band
- Alcohol or betadine preparation

To place a saline lock, use the following procedure (Figures 10.2a to 10.2d):

1. Take appropriate BSI precautions.
2. Attach the syringe containing the saline to the medication port of the saline lock.
3. Flush the saline lock with the saline, leaving at least 2 milliliters in the syringe for use later.
4. Select an appropriate site for venipuncture.
5. Place the constricting band approximately 2 inches proximal (above) to the intended site of puncture.
6. Cleanse the venipuncture site with alcohol or betadine preparations.
7. Insert the venipuncture device into the vein as described for a traditional IV.
8. Slide the IV catheter into the vein using the normal procedure.
9. Carefully remove the metal stylet and promptly dispose of it into a needle disposal container (sharps container).

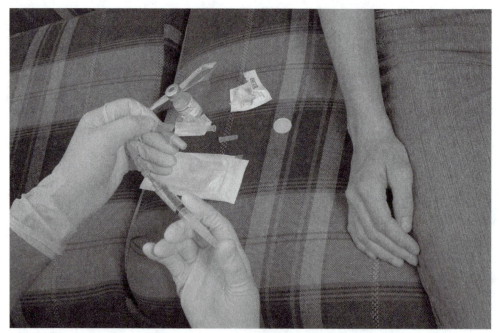

Figure 10.2a. Assemble necessary equipment and flush the saline lock.

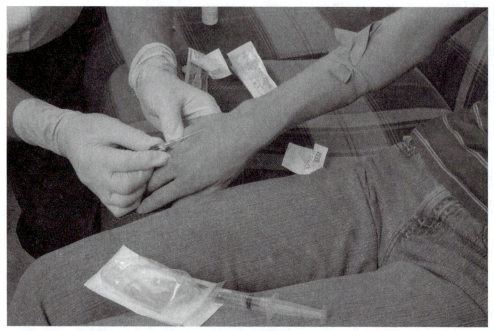

Figure 10.2b. Establish vascular access per normal procedure.

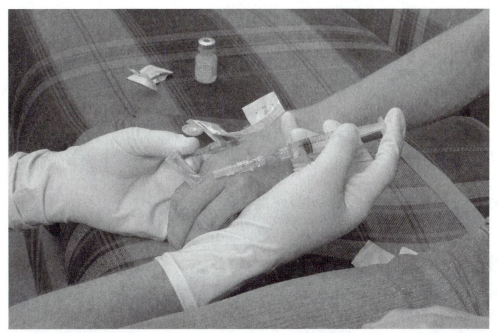

Figure 10.2c. After cannulating the vein and attaching the saline lock, flush lock with 2–3 mL of saline to ensure patency.

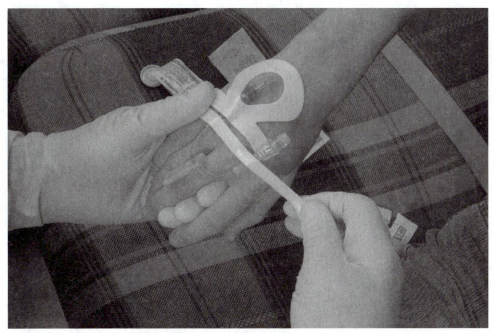

Figure 10.2d. Dress and secure the site using normal procedures.

10. Remove the venous constricting band.

11. Attach the saline lock tubing to the catheter hub.

12. Inject at least 2 milliliters of saline from the syringe into the lock.

13. Secure the catheter and saline lock with tape.

14. Cover the site of puncture with a Band-Aid or commercial membrane.

If the saline is easy to inject into the saline lock and no signs of infiltration or hematoma present, the site is patent. If you encounter resistance when injecting the saline or signs of infiltration become apparent, the site is not patent and the saline lock must be reattempted. Remove the IV catheter as described earlier in this section.

Venous Blood Sampling

On Target

Obtaining venous blood samples when starting the IV is advantageous because this decreases the need in the hospital and saves the patient from experiencing multiple needle sticks. Some EMS systems only obtain venous blood in specific situations. Be sure to follow local protocol.

Venous blood sampling can provide valuable information about the sick or injured patient. Concentrations of electrolytes, gases, hormones, or other chemicals in blood can often shed light on the underlying cause(s) of a patient's complaint. Venous blood is commonly obtained at the same time an IV is started, using the IV catheter to draw the blood. Therefore, in many EMS systems, health care providers placing an IV simultaneously obtain venous blood samples. Doing so saves considerable hospital time and avoids multiple needle sticks for the patient. However, you should never stop to draw blood if it will delay critical aspects of patient care. Consider also that venous blood sampling is best done with a needle gauge of 18 or larger. Smaller sizes can be used but run a higher risk of damaging red blood cells during the blood sampling, rendering the acquisition useless.

If your system allows EMTs to obtain venous blood samples, you will need the following equipment:

On Target

It is critical that the EMT fill the blood tubes in the correct order. Failure to do so may contaminate the blood or result in other problems that will render the drawn blood useless for laboratory analysis.

- **Blood Tubes. Blood tubes** are glass or plastic tubes used to obtain and store the patient's blood. Blood tubes have color-coded, self-healing rubber tops and come in different sizes. Blood tubes for adults generally hold 5 to 7 milliliters of blood, whereas blood tubes for pediatrics hold 2 to 3 milliliters. Blood tubes are vacuum packed, and many contain an anticoagulant that keeps the blood from clotting once in the tube. Blood tubes have an expiration date and must not be used after the date has passed (Figure 10.3).

  Filling blood tubes in their correct order is essential. Blood tubes have different colored tops to allow a quick visual identification of what blood values could be taken from that sample. Different blood tubes may or may not have an additive inside to mix with the blood that will be stored inside until the testing occurs. The EMT must be cognizant to the fact that because of the additives, there is a prescribed order in which the blood tubes should be filled. Not following the proper sequence when filling the blood tubes can skew laboratory tests performed on the blood in the hospital. Always follow local protocol for the order in which blood tubes should be filled.

- **Blood Tube Holder and Luer Lock.** The **blood tube holder** is commonly referred to as a **vacutainer**. A special adapter called a **luer lock**

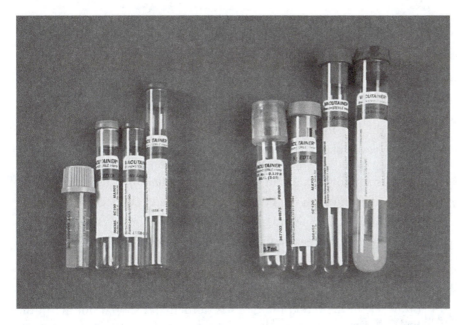

Figure 10.3.
Various blood sampling tubes for adults and pediatrics.

fits into the tube holder. The luer lock contains a rubber-covered needle that punctures the self-healing top of the blood tube once inserted into the tube holder. The remaining portion of the luer lock protrudes from the tube holder and fits snugly into the hub of the IV catheter (Figure 10.4).

Figure 10.4. Vacutainer hub and luer lock adapter (unassembled) are commonly used when obtaining venous blood samples.

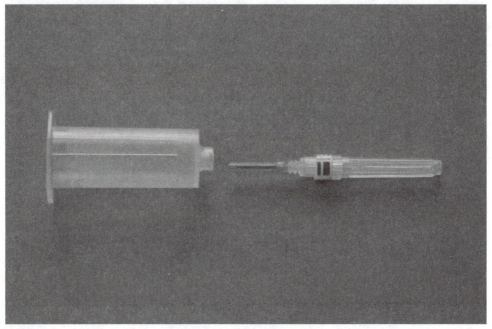

Occasionally, you may be required to obtain blood from an already placed IV catheter. This should be done prior to any medication administration. For this procedure, use the following guidelines (Figures 10.5a to 10.5e):

1. Assemble and prepare all equipment. Inspect the blood tubes for expiration or damage.
2. Insert the luer lock into the blood tube holder (vacutainer).

   Note: Never place blood tubes into the assembled vacutainer and luer lock until you are ready to draw blood. The premature puncture will destroy the vacuum in the blood tube, making it useless.
3. Access the vein with the IV catheter, but do not connect IV tubing.
4. Instead, insert the luer adapter into the hub of the IV catheter.
5. Insert the blood tubes (see Table 10.1 for the correct order in which to use the blood tubes) into the blood tube holder so the rubber-covered needle of the luer lock punctures the self-healing rubber top.
6. Allow blood to enter and fill each tube. There may be a small amount of air left in the blood tube, this is normal and should not alarm the EMT. If no blood enters the blood tube, then the catheter is improperly placed or the blood tube has lost its vacuum.
7. Gently invert the tubes to mix the anticoagulant and the blood the specified number of times (Table 10.1).

Figure 10.5a. **Assemble equipment by securing the luer lock adapter into the vacutainer hub.**

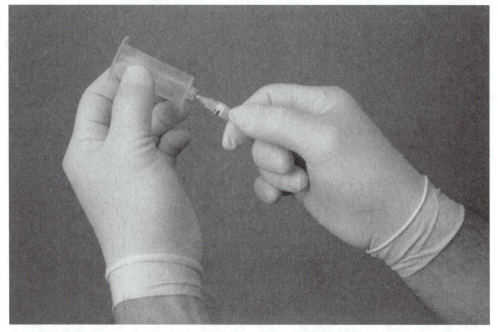

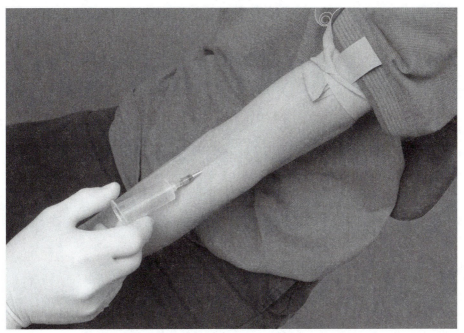

Figure 10.5b. Attach the vacutainer assembly to the hub of the IV catheter.

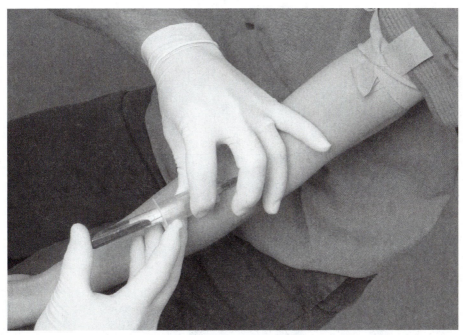

Figure 10.5c. Secure device with one hand while carefully engaging blood tube. Allow blood tube to fill.

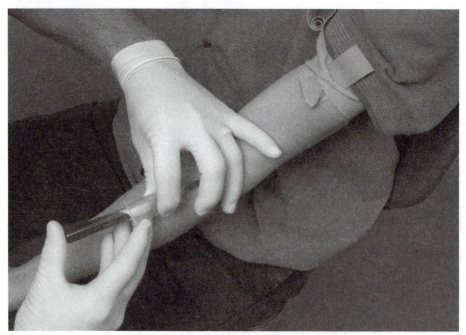

Figure 10.5d. Keep blood tube engaged until tube fills with blood.

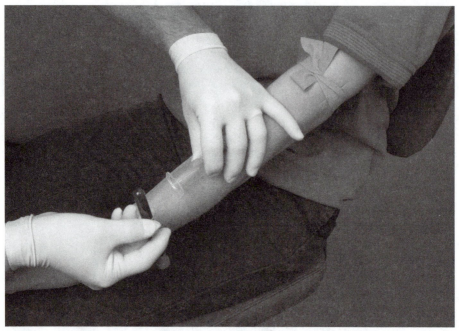

Figure 10.5e. After disengaging filled blood tube, invert it as appropriate (never shake the blood tube).

Table 10.1. **Correct Order for Blood Tubes**

Draw Order	Color of Top (stopper)	Additive	Number of Inversions
1	Red	None	0
2	Blue	Citrate	8
3	Green	Saline	8
4	Purple (lavender)	EDTA	8
5	Gray	Fluoride	8

8. Remove the blood tube holder and luer lock from the hub of the IV catheter and attach the IV tubing.

9. Ensure patency by administering several milliliters of IV fluid.

10. Secure the IV as previously described and set the proper flow rate.

11. Dispose of the luer lock and vacutainer hub in an appropriate biohazard container.

12. Label all blood tubes with the following information:

- Patient's first and last name
- Patient's age and gender
- Date and time drawn
- Name and EMS service of the person drawing the blood

Some EMS systems also employ a "blood band" for stricter matching of the blood sample with the patient. This system employs a bracelet that has adhesive stickers printed with a unique identification number. On this band, you would write the same information as previously listed, attach the band to the patient's wrist, and then attach one of the ID stickers to each blood tube.

If commercial equipment is not available, a 20-milliliter syringe (without a hypodermic needle attached) can be attached to the hub of the IV catheter. Once attached to the IV catheter, pull the plunger back so blood accumulates in the barrel of the syringe. When the syringe is full, remove it from the IV catheter and attach the IV administration tubing. Carefully attach a hypodermic needle to the syringe to puncture the tops of the blood tubes and fill them with the blood. This should occur in the appropriate order. When finished, properly dispose of all needles in a needle disposal container. Finish by labeling the blood tubes.

Complications from drawing blood include damage to the vein wall, inadvertent removal of the IV catheter, and hemolysis (destruction of red blood cells). When red blood cells are destroyed, they release hemoglobin, rendering the blood unusable. The most common causes of hemolysis are vigorously shaking the blood tubes once the blood has been placed inside or using too small of a needle for retrieval (generally no smaller than a 18–20 gauge catheter).

On Target

Failure to properly label the blood tubes causes confusion to which patient it belongs to and will result in the hospital discarding the blood.

On Target

Obtaining blood with a syringe and hypodermic needle increases the EMT's risk for an accidental needle stick. When possible, use a luer lock or syringe without the hypodermic needle as described.

It is important to remember that the circulating volume of an infant or young child is much less than that of an adult. Children can be adversely affected by small amounts of blood loss. Therefore, if obtaining a venous specimen, take the smallest amount of blood possible.

Case Study Follow-Up

You are transporting a 46-year-old female who suffered a serious laceration to her right hand. She is being transferred to a medical facility approximately 2 hours away for specialized surgery and rehabilitative services. An IV of 0.9% NSS was established by hospital personnel in her left forearm with a 16-gauge catheter. The IV has been running at a rate between TKO and WO. During transport, you realize that the IV fluid bag is almost empty. Because it will be another 45 minutes before you arrive at the receiving facility, you must hang a new bag of IV fluid.

To change the IV fluid bag, you retrieve a new bag of 1,000 milliliters of 0.9% NSS. Inspection of the bag reveals it to be in date and free of any particulate or other contaminates. After applying a new pair of gloves, you remove the protective cap over the administration set port. While holding the new bag of IV fluid in your nondominant hand, you close the slide clamp on the existing administration tubing so the flow of IV fluid through the existing IV is stopped. The old bag of fluid is removed from the administration tubing and the spike inserted into the new bag. You ensure the drip chamber is filled appropriately and reopen the slide clamp. The new IV fluid begins to flow into the patient at the previous rate. You document the change of the IV bag and the total volume infused en route to the second destination. The remainder of the trip is uneventful, and the patient does well in surgery.

■ SUMMARY

There may be times when you will have to perform special procedures related to IV therapy such as removing a nonfunctional IV, along with changing the bag of IV fluids or administration tubing after the IV has already been established. Some EMS systems may also permit the EMT to obtain venous blood samples or place a saline lock instead of a more traditional IV. All these procedures are important and require the EMT to employ specific techniques to ensure the patient does not suffer any undue complications. Doing so further enhances the EMT's ability to provide IV therapy and augment the care provided to the sick or injured patient.

REVIEW QUESTIONS

1. An IV that is infiltrated is nonfunctional and must be removed.
   A. True
   B. False

2. Which of the following steps must be performed when changing a fluid bag on an existing IV?
   A. Remove the administration tubing from the empty IV bag.
   B. Attach a syringe to evacuate all fluid from the tubing prior to removing it from the IV catheter.
   C. Remove the IV catheter from the patient prior to replacing the tubing.
   D. Restart the IV on the patient's other extremity.

3. If required to change the IV administration tubing after the IV has already been established, the EMT must
   A. restart the IV.
   B. insert a new IV catheter with the new administration tubing attached.
   C. attach the new IV tubing to the medication port located on the IV tubing already in place.
   D. detach the existing IV tubing from the hub of the catheter and insert the new tubing.

4. A saline lock differs from a more traditional IV setup in that it
   A. uses a larger IV catheter than a traditional IV setup.
   B. does not contain a bag of IV fluid.
   C. uses a smaller IV catheter than a traditional IV setup.
   D. does not require the EMT to use sterile precautions when placing the lock.

5. Drawing blood at the same time an IV is started is beneficial because it
   A. allows the EMT to better diagnose the patient's problem.
   B. saves the patient from multiple needle sticks.
   C. permits the EMT to determine whether the IV has been accidentally placed in an artery.
   D. can be injected into the IV fluid bag to make a blood solution.

6. Blood tubes have an expiration date and should not be used if expired.
   A. True
   B. False

7. Which of the following represents the best technique for removing the IV catheter from an infiltrated IV site?
   A. Have a physician remove the catheter with forceps.
   B. Swiftly remove the catheter by pulling straight back.
   C. Remove the catheter by first removing the hub with scissors and then pulling back on the remaining Teflon.
   D. Cut the hub of the catheter with scissors.

8. To determine whether a saline lock is patent, you would
   A. attach a syringe and withdraw at least 10 mL of blood.
   B. allow approximately 10 mL of IV fluid to flow from the IV fluid bag into the patient.
   C. inject at least 2 mL of normal saline solution into the lock.
   D. not need to determine patency because saline locks are not placed in a vein.

9. Changing the IV administration tubing on an IV that is already established is a sterile process.
   A. True
   B. False

10. To obtain venous blood samples, the EMT should
    A. draw blood from the medication administration port of the IV tubing.
    B. collect blood in a 10-mL syringe and then pour it into the blood tubes whose tops have been previously removed.
    C. use a special blood collection IV catheter when starting the IV.
    D. draw blood from the IV catheter prior to connecting the administration tubing.

Legal Concerns and Documentation

LEARNING OBJECTIVES

By the end of this chapter, you should be able to:

- ☑ Discuss how the EMT scope of practice affects the EMT's ability to provide IV therapy, including acts of omission and commission
- ☑ Discuss how patient consent affects IV therapy
- ☑ Describe how acts of assault and battery related to IV therapy can lead to liability for the EMT
- ☑ Describe negligence and how it can lead to areas of liability related to IV therapy
- ☑ Discuss the importance of documentation related to IV therapy
- ☑ List important information that must be documented for routine IV therapy, unsuccessful attempts, complications, and refusal of IV treatment

---

KEY WORDS

Abandonment—The termination of the EMT–patient relationship without providing for the appropriate continuation of care at the same or higher level.

Assault—Any act that unlawfully places a person in apprehension of bodily harm without his or her consent.

Battery—The physical touching of a patient without his or her consent.

Commission—Any act or intervention in which the EMT goes beyond his or her scope of practice or was performed when it was inappropriate to do so.

Consent—The granting of permission to treat. Consent is based on the idea that every adult who is of sound mind and able to make informed decisions has the right to determine what should be done regarding his or her medical care.

Expressed consent—Consent obtained when the patient directly grants permission for treatment, either verbally, nonverbally, or in writing.

Implied consent—The idea that any patient unable to make sound decisions regarding his or her care would provide expressed consent if able to do so.

Informed consent—Consent granted by the patient based on full disclosure of information, including benefits, risks, and danger of refusing care.

Involuntary consent—Consent to treat ordered by the authority of a court, even though the patient may not want it.

Negligence—Harm that is attributable to improper actions of the EMT. Negligence is the single greatest area of potential liability for the EMT related to IV therapy.

Omission—Failure of the EMT to provide a particular aspect(s) of care that is warranted.

PCR—Prehospital care report. Sometimes also referred to as a "trip sheet" or a "run sheet."

Scope of practice—A formal description of what EMTs are allowed and expected to perform. Typically, the scope of practice is established by state law or by the local medical director.

Case Study

You have just arrived at work and are headed to the locker room to change when the shift supervisor calls you to his office. He asks you to sit down and begins to explain that a patient you treated 6 months ago has filed a lawsuit, involving the hospital, the EMS system, and you. Apparently, the IV you initiated in the field became dislodged, causing massive infiltration and swelling to the patient's arm, which ultimately resulted in permanent neurological damage, and the person now only has limited use of the extremity. Because the call occurred 6 months ago and you function in a high-volume EMS system, you have difficulty remembering the exact call. How will you proceed?

Chapter 11 discusses areas of legal liability related to IV therapy. The importance of documentation and examples of proper documentation are also presented. At the end of the chapter, we return to this case and apply your knowledge.

QUESTIONS

1. What is the most important piece of information related to this accusation that has been documented in the PCR?

2. What may have happened if the EMT did not thoroughly document the IV therapy provided?

3. Given the information in the case study, and assuming IV therapy is within the EMT's scope of practice, could the EMT also be accused of an act of commission or omission?

■ INTRODUCTION

The addition of IV therapy to the EMT scope of practice represents a significant step forward in caring for the sick and the injured. However, such an addition comes with increased responsibility, especially that related to legal concerns and documentation. As an EMT empowered to provide IV therapy, you are expected to do so in a safe and effective manner. You are responsible for any and all complications that result from the IV and ensuing therapy, as well as any complications that may arise. To avoid incurring unnecessary liability, the EMT must be aware of areas of potential liability and properly document all information related to the IV therapy. This may be the only means of defense if something goes wrong.

Legal Concerns Related to IV Therapy

The EMT should be aware of the following legal topics when rendering IV therapy in the prehospital setting.

Scope of Practice. The range of duties and skills EMTs are allowed and expected to perform is called the scope of practice. Typically, the **scope of practice** is established by state law and may also be influenced by the local medical director. The EMT can only provide IV therapy if it is contained within his or her scope of practice. If IV therapy is not contained within the scope of practice and the EMT performs the intervention, he or she will face serious discipline, most likely resulting in the revocation of certification. Therefore, to provide IV therapy as an EMT, it must first be written into the EMT's scope of practice.

> **On Target**
>
> If IV therapy is not included in the EMT's scope of practice, he or she cannot legally provide this care.

Practicing above or below the scope of practice can expose the EMT to charges of omission and commission:

- **Omission.** An act of **omission** describes failure of the EMT to provide a specific act or treatment given a particular set of circumstances. For instance, neglecting to attempt an IV on a patient with chest pain when the standard of care dictates that patients with chest pain are to receive IV therapy may be viewed as an act of omission. Using equipment that is not indicated for the clinical presentation may also constitute an act of omission. For example, providing IV therapy with a microdrip administration set for a person requiring massive fluid infusion might be interpreted as an act of omission.

  Generally, for legal action to be taken, the patient must incur some sort of harm secondary to the act of omission. For instance, if an IV is not attempted on a patient with chest pain and the patient goes into cardiac arrest and dies because medications could not be administered in a timely manner by ALS personnel, an act of omission may be present.

When harm does occur, the act of omission translates into negligence (discussed later). However, even if harm does not occur, the system medical director may take remedial or disciplinary measures for two reasons. First, the EMT has performed incorrectly. Second, this exposes the medical director and his or her license to unnecessary liability.

- **Commission.** An act of **commission** refers to the EMT going beyond his or her scope of practice. As mentioned previously, providing IV therapy when this practice is not included in the EMT's scope of practice would constitute an act of commission. Starting an IV in the scalp of a pediatric when local and/or state medical guidelines stipulate that the EMT cannot use this site is another example of commission. Likewise, administering a medication through an IV line when practice is not allowed would be an allegation of an act of commission.

The key to avoiding liability from acts of omission or commission is familiarity with scope of practice and not acting above or below these measures. This does not only apply to IV therapy, but to all aspects of prehospital care provided by the EMT. If extenuating circumstances exist, contact medical direction and/or document thoroughly.

Consent. By law, you must obtain a patient's consent prior to providing any medical care or transport. **Consent** is the granting of permission to treat and is based on the idea that every adult who is of sound mind and able to make informed decisions has the right to determine what should be done regarding his or her medical care.

The best kind of consent is informed consent. **Informed consent** describes consent granted by the patient based on full disclosure of information, in this case, the benefits and risks related to IV therapy, as well as the danger of refusing an IV. Prior to starting an IV, informed consent must be obtained from every and all competent adults. Adult is defined as 18 years of age or older in most states. For those younger than 18 years of age, a child's parent or legal guardian must provide informed consent prior to treatment, including IV therapy (exceptions include emancipated minors such as those who are pregnant, have children, or are financially independent and living away from home). Consent can be categorized into the following:

- **Expressed Consent. Expressed consent** occurs when the patient directly grants permission for treatment either verbally, nonverbally, or in writing after being provided with the risks and benefits of treatment (in this case, IV therapy).

- **Implied Consent.** When a minor (younger than 18 years of age) requires IV therapy and a parent or guardian is not present, treatment can be given under the premise of **implied consent** (assuming the IV therapy is indicated). Implied consent (also referred to as "emergency doctrine") states that the patient's parent or legal guardian would want the IV therapy performed and would provide consent to do so if they were present. The same holds true for an adult patient who is sick or injured to the point where he or she cannot make sound decisions regarding his or her care. An example would be a trauma patient in shock who is

On Target

To avoid committing an act of omission or commission, the EMT should be familiar with exactly what he or she is required to do and never deviate above or below this standard. If extenuating circumstances exist, precise documentation is critical.

On Target

Except for a very few circumstances, consent from the patient is required prior to starting or providing IV therapy. Failure to gain consent places the EMT in a position of increased legal liability.

On Target

The best form of consent is expressed consent.

confused and not able to communicate adequately. Again, the premise of implied consent states that the patient would consent to IV therapy if he or she were able to do so.

- **Involuntary Consent. Involuntary consent** describes treatment ordered by the authority of a court, even though the patient may not want it. Involuntary consent is most frequently encountered for patients who are being held for mental health or behavioral issues. The EMT may be called on to provide care to such individuals, up to and including IV therapy.

Failure to obtain appropriate consent before establishing an IV can result in serious legal problems for the EMT, particularly in the areas of assault and battery:

- **Assault. Assault** describes an act that unlawfully places a person in apprehension of bodily harm without his consent. For example, consider the patient who is scared of needles and refuses IV therapy. Showing the patient the sharp venipuncture device and placing it on his or her arm as if to start an IV may leave the EMT open to charges of assault.

- **Battery. Battery** is defined as the physical touching of a patient without his or her consent. For a patient who is alert, oriented, and 18 years of age or older, starting an IV without first gaining his or her consent to do so may be the basis for battery. For a minor or incapacitated adult, failure to gain consent from the appropriate parent, family member, or legal guardian can also result in the accusation of battery.

  If IV therapy is required for a minor and a responsible party cannot be located, it is acceptable to provide IV therapy under the auspices of implied consent (assuming IV therapy is indicated). The same holds true for any individual with a decreased level of consciousness or anyone else incapable of making decisions for him- or herself.

To avoid allegations such as assault and battery, always gain the patient's or responsible party's expressed consent prior to starting an IV. If the patient or legal guardian refuses the IV therapy, make several attempts to persuade him or her to allow you to start the IV by explaining how it will benefit him or her. If the patient or legal guardian still refuses, document accordingly (discussed later) and/or contact medical direction for advisement.

A competent adult, parent, or legal guardian may withdraw consent for any reason at any time. This even includes IV therapy after consent was initially obtained. When this situation is encountered, make several attempts to persuade him or her to allow you to start the IV by explaining how it will benefit him or her. If the consent cannot be reobtained, document accordingly (discussed later) and/or contact medical direction for advisement.

Negligence. As an EMT, you are required to administer IV therapy consistent with your education and training and equal to that of any other EMT with equivalent training. You are also expected to perform IV therapy in a reasonable and prudent manner, as would another EMT given

On Target

If a minor or critically ill or injured adult patient who is unable to provide consent due to his or her injuries requires IV therapy, the EMT can legally provide such care under the protection of implied consent.

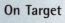

On Target

To avoid allegations such as assault and battery, always gain the patient's or responsible party's expressed consent prior to starting an IV.

a similar situation. Failure to do so may result in allegations of **negligence** (sometimes referred to as "malpractice").

Negligence related to IV therapy is the single greatest area of potential liability for the EMT. Negligence occurs when the patient incurs some sort of harm or damage that is attributable to actions of the EMT. In a negligence claim related to IV therapy, the patient or other party making the allegation must establish and prove four elements:

1. **Duty to Act.** The EMT has a formal or legal obligation to provide IV therapy in a safe and/or prudent manner.

2. **Breach of Duty.** The EMT did not provide IV therapy in a safe and/or prudent manner, or as other EMTs with equivalent training and education would, usually by an act of omission or commission.

3. **Actual Damages.** The patient incurred harm or injury related to the IV therapy.

4. **Proximate Cause.** The EMT's actions related to the IV therapy directly caused the injury or harm incurred by the patient.

IV therapy is an invasive procedure that if not performed properly can result in harm or injury. If in a court of law, these four components of negligence are shown to be present, then the EMT can be held liable for the harm incurred by the patient. This obviously leaves the EMT with significant legal problems. Specific situations that may lead to allegations of negligence include the following:

On Target

Negligence related to IV therapy is the single greatest area of potential liability for the EMT. For negligence to be proven, the patient must incur some sort of damage caused by improper action or inaction on behalf of the EMT.

- **Omission or Commission.** As previously discussed, harm resulting from acts of omission or commission may result in charges of negligence.

- **Equipment Defect/Malfunction.** The EMT may be accountable for harm resulting from defective equipment if he or she does not inspect the materials and supplies prior to use. For example, a localized or systemic infection resulting from the use of nonsterile or contaminated materials may result in a negligent claim directed toward the EMT. A pyrogenic reaction caused by using contaminated IV fluid can result in legal action against the EMT because proper technique indicates that inspection of the solution should have occurred prior to use. Using the proper technique and inspecting all materials prior to use provide the best defense against negligence related to equipment defect and malfunction.

- **Complications.** Complications that result from IV therapy may be legally viewed as "harm" and a source of liability for the EMT. (See Chapter 7 for a discussion of complications related to IV therapy.) If the complication(s) can be attributed to the EMT's actions in starting and/or maintaining the IV, legal action may result.

  A complication(s) resulting from poor technique when starting the IV or use of an inappropriate site may be the source of a negligent claim. For example, an infection resulting from the EMT's failure to prepare the site with alcohol or betadine prior to catheter insertion, or puncture and damage of a tendon or nerve with resultant injury are examples of potential negligence. Swelling and pain caused by placing an IV in the arm of a patient who has had a breast removed on the same side may also predispose the EMT to negligence. A fragment that breaks free from the IV catheter device and lodges in the lungs as a result of improper insertion technique provides yet another area of negligence.

Using proper technique and materials and choosing the most appropriate site, along with following local medical guidelines when providing IV therapy, are the best defenses against harmful complications and potential negligence.

Abandonment. **Abandonment** is the termination of the EMT–patient relationship without providing for the appropriate continuation of care while it is still needed or desired by the patient. Once an EMT has initiated an IV, he or she must ensure any and all care is transferred to medical personnel with the same or greater privileges or abilities related to IV therapy (e.g., another EMT able to provide IV therapy, or an EMT–Intermediate, paramedic, or prehospital registered nurse). In the field or during transport, it would be inappropriate for the EMT to establish an IV and then turn care over to another EMT who has not been vested with the same IV privileges. In the hospital, leaving the patient with an IV in the care of someone other than a physician or nurse may also open the EMT up to charges of abandonment.

Documentation and IV Therapy. Documentation is a critical aspect of IV therapy and must be considered just as important as the actual placement and maintenance of the IV. Formal documentation is the only record as to the care and events that transpired. As such, documentation may be the only form of protection should a complaint or complication related to the IV arise at a later time. Proper documentation of IV therapy serves many purposes:

- Proof that an IV(s) was initiated
- A record of the medical treatment administered by EMS
- Status of the IV throughout transport and transfer of care
- A record of supplies and materials used
- Information for billing and reimbursement
- Quality assurance information
- Research data

As with all other documentation related to prehospital care, the information recorded must be objective, thorough, and truthful. As the saying goes, "If it is not written down, it was not done."

Basic IV Documentation. Information related to IV therapy must be recorded in the **PCR.** The format of PCRs varies from system to system, as does the way that information is documented. Some PCRs entail that the EMT check pertinent boxes, fill in bubbles, write free narrative, or a combination there of. Some EMS systems use computerized charting.

On Target

To avoid charges of abandonment after placing an IV, only turn patient care over to another EMT, EMT–Intermediate, paramedic, nurse, or physician after providing an oral update as to the patients condition.

On Target

Documentation is a critical aspect of IV therapy and considered the only formal record of treatment. Documentation may be the EMT's only source of protection if legal action is taken at a later time.

Regardless of the format, the following information must be placed, as a minimum, on the PCR:

- **Initiation of the IV.** After initiating an IV, the following information should be documented in the PCR:
  - Name of person(s) initiating IV
  - Time of IV initiation
  - Specific site (e.g., right/left hand, right/left forearm, right/left AC region)
  - Gauge and length of IV catheter
  - Type of IV administration tubing
  - Solution (type, container size, and number of bags, if more than one, used)
  - IV flow rate administered
  - Method to protect site
  - Total number of successful and unsuccessful attempts (if any)
  - Related complications (if any)

Consider the following examples:

"IV initiated with 18 G/1" catheter, macrodrip administration tubing, 500 mL 0.9% NSS in (R) hand by C. Demmings—EMT (1600). (+) Patency. Site covered and secured with tape and protective membrane. No complications observed. IV infused at a KVO rate."

Initiation of IV	
Time	16:00
Person initiating IV	Demmings, EMT
Gauge/length	18 G/1"
Administration tubing	Macrodrop (10 gtts/mL)
Type/Volume of solution	0.9% NSS/500 mL
Patency	Ⓨ N
Site protection	Tape/Tegraderm
Complications	None
Successful/Unsuccessful	1/0
Infusion rate	KVO

- **Maintenance of the IV.** For IV maintenance after it has been established, include the following information on the PCR:
  - Patency of IV
  - Flow rate(s) of IV solution if altered from initial setting (e.g., you decide to give a fluid bolus at a WO rate due to the patient's condition)

- Patient response to IV therapy
- Related complications

Consider the following example:

"IV patent throughout prehospital care. 40 mL bolus of 0.9% NSS followed by TKO rate during transport. No change in patient condition secondary to IV therapy. No complications observed."

- **Status of the IV When Transferring Care.** After transferring care of a patient with an IV, include the following information in the PCR:
  - Person and title to which IV and overall patient care was transferred
  - Time of transfer of care
  - Patency of IV at time of transfer
  - Condition of IV site at time of transfer
  - Flow rate at time of transfer
  - Number of milliliters of solution administered
  - Number of milliliters remaining in IV solution container

Consider the following examples:

"Patient care transferred to J. Shuman, RN, @ 1620. IV patent, site showing no abnormalities, TKO rate at time of transfer. Total of 60 mL of 0.9% NSS administered/540 mL remaining in bag."

IV Therapy/Transfer of Care	
Time	16:20
Person assuming care	J. Shuman, RN
IV patent	Ⓨ N
Site condition	(−) Abnormalities
Flow rate	TKO
Milliliters administered	60 mL
Milliliters remaining	440 mL

On Target

Not only should documentation describe the initiation of the IV, but also the maintenance and status of the IV when the patient is transferred to another health care provider.

Although it seems like this is a lot of information to place in the PCR, you must realize that this may be the only record of the care provided after the call is complete. Therefore, for your protection and for the purposes listed previously, it is essential that you thoroughly document these aspects of IV therapy in the PCR. Figure 11.1 shows one approach to documentation as it appears on the EMS PCR.

The EMT must remember that a patient on whom he or she established an IV may be passed to several different health care providers and/or moved through different areas of the hospital for tests and care. In the process, there are opportunities for dislodgment of the IV, infection of the site, inappropriate changes in flow rate, original fluids changed to inappropriate fluids, and so forth. To avoid facing undue blame or legal difficulties for problems caused by others, it is critical that the EMT take the time to

Figure 11.1.
Typical portion of PCR where information regarding IV access is documented.

IV THERAPY -- IV #1		
SUCCESSFUL Y N # OF ATTEMPTS _____		
ANGIO SIZE _____ga.		
SITE _____		
TOTAL FLUID INFUSED _____CC		
BLOOD DRAW Y N INITIALS _____		
IV THERAPY -- IV #2		
SUCCESSFUL Y N # OF ATTEMPTS _____		
ANGIO SIZE _____ga.		
SITE _____		
TOTAL FLUID INFUSED _____CC		
BLOOD DRAW Y N INITIALS _____		

thoroughly document the information as presented. This may very well be the only protection afforded to the EMT if something goes wrong after transferring care of the patient.

Special Situations Requiring Additional Documentation. There are several situations that require additional documentation. These include the following:

- **Unsuccessful Attempts.** It is more difficult to start an IV on some persons than on others. There will be times that, despite appropriate technique, an IV cannot be established initially. Even though the IV was not successfully placed, it must still be documented. When an IV is unsuccessful, record the following information in the PCR:
  - Name of person(s) initiating IV
  - Time of IV initiation
  - Specific site (e.g., right/left hand, right/left forearm, right/left AC region)
  - Gauge and length of IV catheter
  - Reason IV was considered unsuccessful (e.g., infiltration, no flashback, unable to thread catheter, no flow of solution)
  - Removal of intact catheter
  - Control of hemorrhage and/or method to protect site after removal

  Consider the following example:

  "IV initiated with 18 G/1" catheter/macrodrip administration tubing, 500 mL 0.9% NSS in (R) hand by C. Demmings—EMT

(1600). IV infiltrates with introduction of fluid. IV catheter removed intact. Pressure dressing applied. Hemorrhage controlled/site covered with sterile dressing and bandage."

- **Complications from IV Therapy.** Even with perfect technique and proper procedure, complications from IV therapy may arise. (Review Chapter 7 for complications related to IV therapy.) If a complication related to the IV occurs while in your care, do not cover it up by not documenting its occurrence. Rather, objectively document the complication and the method or care taken to remedy or treat the situation. Never hide or falsify information related to a complication. It must be remembered that IV therapy contains the potential for complications despite appropriate technique.

Consider the following example:

"After placement of the IV, the patient displayed a sudden onset of hives and itching. Allergic reaction suspected. IV catheter removed intact, and site cleaned with alcohol and covered with sterile gauze and tape. Medical direction (Dr. Cole) contacted for advisement. . ."

Some complications may occur hours to days after you started the IV. In such cases, your only course of defense is the documentation in the PCR. To avoid taking blame for a complication(s) that may very well be the responsibility of another, take the time to thoroughly document all information related to initiation of the IV.

> **On Target**
> Never attempt to hide unsuccessful IV attempts or complications that occur in relation to the IV therapy!

- **Refusal of IV Therapy.** Special documentation is required when a patient refuses IV therapy. Any competent adult or parent or legal guardian of a minor has a legal right to refuse care or part of that care, including IV therapy. If a patient refuses IV therapy, make several attempts to persuade him or her to receive the treatment. Inform the patient why you want to start an IV and the potential consequences of refusing. If the patient still refuses, carefully document the following information to avoid potential legal problems:

  - Why patient needed the IV therapy
  - Whether the patient (or parent/legal guardian) is an adult with full mental capacity (alert and oriented)
  - Number of attempts made to persuade the patient to accept the IV therapy
  - Whether patient was informed of potential consequences of not receiving IV therapy
  - Whether patient knowing and willingly signed a refusal of service related to the IV

"Patient required IV therapy due to chest pain. Patient refused IV therapy due to bad experience in the past with IVs. EMS made three attempts to get patient to consent to IV therapy. Patient informed of potential medical consequences by not accepting the IV therapy; the patient stated he understood these consequences, but still refused to give consent. EMS explained need to sign a

Figure 11.2.
Portion of PCR showing the refusal of treatment area that must be completed if the patient declines the EMT's care.

RELEASE FROM RESPONSIBILITY

DATE _____ 19 _____ TIME _____ a.m. / p.m.

This is to certify that _____

is refusing   ☐ TREATMENT   ☐ TRANSPORTATION

against the advice of the attending Emergency Medical Technician and of the Phoenix Fire Department, and when applicable, the base hospital and the base hospital physician.

I acknowledge that I have been informed of the following:

1. The nature and potential of the illness or injuries.
2. The potential risks of delaying treatment and transportation, up to and including death.
3. The availability of ambulance transportation to a hospital for treatment.

Nevertheless, I assume all risks and consequences of my decision, including further physical deterioration, loss of limb, paralysis, and even death, and hereby release the attending Emergency Medical Technician and the Phoenix Fire Department, and when applicable, the base hospital and the base hospital physician from any ill effects which may result from my refusal.

Witness _____   Signed: **X** _____

Witness _____   Relationship to Patient _____

Refusal must be signed by the patient; or by the nearest relative or legal guardian in the case of a minor, or when patient is physically or mentally incompetent.

☐ Patient refuses to sign release despite efforts of attending Emergency Medical Technician to obtain such signature after informing patient of concerns listed in numbers 1, 2, and 3 above.

GUIDELINES — Patient Refusal Documentation

In addition to those items normally documented (chief complaint, history of present illness, mechanism of injury, physical assessment, etc.) the following items should be recorded, regardless of patient's cooperation:

- Mental Status (orientation, speech, etc.)
- Suspected presence of alcohol or drugs
- Patient's exact words (as much as possible) in the refusal of care OR the signing of the release form
- Circumstances or reasons (including exact words of patient, if possible) for INCOMPLETE ADVISEMENT (risk of injury, abusiveness, unruliness, risk of injury other than from patient, etc.)
- Advice given to patients' guardian(s)

On Target

Because of the increased risk for legal action associated with those who refuse IV therapy, the EMT must ensure he or she makes the patient aware of the risks of refusing and documents this accordingly.

---

refusal for IV therapy. Patient signs informed consent (signature below). Witnessed by family member (signature below). Medical direction notified."

Medical direction can often be a useful resource in such situations and should be used by the EMT as needed. Often, if possible, the physician will talk directly to the patient via phone and convince the patient to cooperate with the EMT care plan. If however, it is impossible to obtain the necessary consent, it is best to get another person, preferably family or friend, to witness a patient's refusal, and then finally you also sign the refusal form. Figure 11.2 shows a patient refusal form (often, the description of the event surrounding the refusal is documented above this space).

Case Study Follow-Up

You have just arrived at work and are headed to the locker room to change when your shift supervisor informs you that a lawsuit has been filed concerning your treatment of a patient 6 months ago. Specifically, the lawsuit alleges negligence related to unrecognized infiltration of the IV and subsequent loss of function to the patient's arm in which the IV was placed.

You and the supervisor retrieve the PCR for the call and review it. At the time, you documented initiation of an IV in the left forearm using a 20-gauge IV catheter, macrodrip tubing, and 500 milliliters of 0.9% NSS. The documentation states that the IV was run at a TKO rate throughout the prehospital phase of care and a total of 15 milliliters of fluid administered. The PCR reads that the IV was patent and running at a TKO rate when transferred to the registered nurse in the emergency department. The specific name of the nurse listed on the PCR and her signature confirms the transfer of patient care.

When comparing the run report with a description of the lawsuit, you notice that the IV in question was in the patient's right arm, not the left. You and your supervisor reason that another IV was placed after prehospital care and transfer of the patient. It was this IV that infiltrated and caused the damage, not the IV you established. The information is passed along to attorneys for both your service and the patient. Several days later, you receive official notice that you and the EMS service have been dismissed from the lawsuit.

Feeling relieved that your documentation was the factor resulting in being dropped from the lawsuit, you ask your supervisor if you can put together a presentation for the service employees describing the need for and benefits of thorough documentation. The presentation is successful, and results in the improvement of documentation for the service overall. Your efforts are noticed by the upper administration, and you are subsequently appointed to the quality assurance committee.

■ SUMMARY

Although IV therapy can be a beneficial medical intervention and greatly advances the EMT's ability to provide care to the sick and injured, it also increases the legal responsibility for the EMT. As an EMT vested with the ability to provide IV therapy, you must do so in a manner that is safe, effective, and beneficial to the patient. The ability to do so and offset the liability associated with IV therapy is easily accomplished by performing IV therapy with the appropriate technique and in accordance with the scope of practice and medical director's guidelines. Thorough documentation is another essential component of IV therapy and must be considered just as important as actual establishment of the IV itself. The result is professional advancement and delivery of unsurpassed patient care.

REVIEW QUESTIONS

1. Which of the following describes battery?
   A. Using an IV fluid that has expired
   B. Starting an IV on a 10-year-old male who does not need an IV
   C. Failure to start an IV when one is clearly indicated
   D. Placing an IV in an alert and oriented adult who refused the IV

2. You are treating a 10-year-old male who has been hit by a car and is in shock. The boy's parents cannot be found. Under what form of consent can you provide IV therapy?
   A. Informed
   B. Expressed
   C. Involuntary
   D. Implied

3. Consent must be obtained any time the EMT initiates an IV.
   A. True
   B. False

4. To avoid the issue of battery, the EMT should
   A. start an IV in all situations.
   B. contact medical direction prior to starting any and all IVs.
   C. contact medical direction prior to providing IV therapy to any patient younger than 18 years of age.
   D. gain the patient's or responsible party's consent.

5. An alert and oriented 46-year-old male patient with cardiac-related chest pain has refused IV therapy. Your next step would be to
   A. have the patient sign a refusal of care form.
   B. explain the benefits of having the IV.
   C. establish the IV against his will.
   D. transport the patient to the hospital.

6. You read about a legal case in which an EMT started an IV on a person in cardiac arrest and then administered a medication through the IV. Although starting an IV was written into the EMT's scope of practice, administering a medication was not. This would be an example of
   A. commission.
   B. duty to act.
   C. abandonment.
   D. omission.

7. Starting an IV is more important than documenting information concerning the IV to the PCR.
   A. True
   B. False

8. Failure to attempt IV therapy on a patient with a decreased level of consciousness when it is written into the EMT protocols by the system medical director could result in the charge of
   A. commission.
   B. battery.

C. abandonment.

D. omission.

9. You are unsuccessful in placing an IV in a patient with chest pain. Consequently, you establish another IV in the opposite arm. In relation to the unsuccessful IV, you should

A. inform the nurse at the emergency department of the unsuccessful IV attempt and document the successful IV.

B. document both the successful and the unsuccessful IV.

C. document the successful IV.

D. inform the physician of the unsuccessful IV and document the successful IV to the PCR.

10. Indicate which of the following items should be included when documenting routine IV therapy by circling YES or NO.

YES   NO   Person and title to which IV and overall patient care was transferred

YES   NO   Time that care was transferred

YES   NO   Patency of IV at time of transfer

YES   NO   Condition of IV site at time of transfer

YES   NO   Flow rate at time of transfer

YES   NO   Number of milliliters of solution administered

YES   NO   Number of milliliters remaining in IV solution container

Case Study Questions
Introduction to IV Therapy

RATIONALES

1. What findings in the initial assessment indicate that the patient is in critical condition?

   The 64-year-old male in this case study has several significant findings that the EMT must recognize as critical. The initial assessment reveals the patient to be confused and bradycardic (heart rate of 32 beats per minute). In addition, the patient is severely hypotensive with a blood pressure of 58/40 mm Hg. Given the scenario, the slow heart rate has resulted in a decreased amount of blood being pumped to the brain, accounting for the altered mental status. By the same token, the heart is incapable of pumping enough blood into the circulatory system to maintain an adequate blood pressure. Collectively, this patient is hemodynamically unstable and must be recognized as critical.

2. Even though the EMT cannot administer the emergency medications that the patient requires, why would starting an IV on the patient be beneficial?

   Although the EMT may not be able to administer the emergency medications required by the patient, establishing an IV is of great benefit. Because the EMT has already established the IV, the nurse(s) in the emergency department will not have to take the time to perform this procedure. Consequently, emergency medications and fluids can be administered without delay as soon as the patient reaches the emergency department.

3. Why would administering medication intravenously to this patient be better than administering the same medication orally?

   Administering medication intravenously to this patient allows the medications to enter the body, become absorbed, and be circulated throughout much faster than if the same medications were administered orally. Also, given the confusion and potential for further demise, it is best not to administer anything by mouth (this decreases the opportunity for aspiration). Because the patient is already vomiting, it is doubtful whether medications administered orally would be retained and therefore be effective.

Anatomy, Physiology, and Mechanism of IV Therapy

RATIONALES

1. Does the fact that the patient is obese raise any concerns or challenges regarding IV therapy?

   Heavy-set people tend to have more subcutaneous fat that those who are not heavy-set. Increased amounts of subcutaneous fat can "bury" veins, making them more difficult to locate for IV therapy. Consequently, placement of an IV in a heavy-set patient can be more challenging than IV placement in those with less body fat.

2. Given the patient's condition, would it matter if the IV were placed in an artery instead of a vein?

   Without exception, IVs are *always* placed in veins and *never* in arteries. The lower blood pressure in veins, along with their thinner walls and closer proximity to the surface of the body, make veins the vessel of choice when providing IV therapy. Accidental puncture of an artery can result in significant hemorrhage that is difficult to control.

3. How would you respond to the patient's question asking how the IV will help him?

   The EMT should inform the patient that he appears to be suffering from an allergic reaction and can benefit from the administration of medications. Establishing an IV will allow these medications to be administered directly into the cardiovascular system, which will enable rapid distribution throughout the body. As a result, the patient will improve faster, as opposed to administering the same medications orally.

4. If the patient asked you whether the IV will hurt, what would you tell him?

   Because the dermal layer of the skin contains pain receptors, most patients feel pain as the sharp IV catheter punctures through the skin and into the vein. However, once the catheter is properly placed in the vein, the patient should no longer feel pain, albeit some may complain of a slight discomfort.

Intravenous Fluid Selection

RATIONALES

1. How might the clinical condition of dehydration affect your ability to locate and access a vein for IV therapy?

   Significant dehydration can decrease the plasma of the blood, therein decreasing the total blood volume. As a result, the veins contain less blood and decrease in size, making them less obvious on the surface of the body. This can affect the EMT's ability to find a suitable vein for IV therapy and access it with the IV catheter. Further compounding the situation is the fact that the body will compensate for a low blood volume by shunting a portion of the remaining blood from the peripheral veins to the larger veins in the core of the body. This makes location and access of peripheral veins even more challenging.

2. Would 5% dextrose in water (D_5W) be an acceptable IV fluid to use for the rehydration of this patient?

   D_5W is not a good fluid for volume replacement and should not be used. Once in the body, the cells rapidly use the glucose contained within the D_5W, leaving only the water. Without the glucose, D_5W becomes a physiologically hypotonic solution, which according to the rules of osmosis, is pulled toward areas containing greater concentrations of electrolytes (the extra vascular space). This results in further depletion of the blood volume as the water is pulled from the vasculature.

3. If 0.9% NSS was not available, what other isotonic crystalloid would be acceptable to use in its place?

   If 0.9% NSS was not available, lactated Ringer's would be the next most appropriate crystalloid. As an isotonic solution, lactated Ringer's would evenly distribute between the intravascular space and cells. Lactated Ringer's also contains some buffering agents that may benefit the dehydrated patient if his or her body pH is altered. The other isotonic crystalloid solution is D_5W, which as described previously, rapidly becomes a hypotonic crystalloid when placed in the body. Accordingly, D_5W is a poor selection for replacing the volume of a dehydrated patient.

Intravenous Site Selection

RATIONALES

1. **What IV fluid would you use for this patient?**

   The most logical choice of IV fluid for this patient would be 0.9% NSS or lactated Ringer's. Of the two isotonic crystalloids, the 0.9% NSS is probably the more commonly used in most EMS systems. Because the patient does not require a large amount of fluid (based on her chief complaint, medical history, and stable vital signs), small amounts of D_5W to keep the vein from clotting off would not be inappropriate. However, most EMS systems reserve D_5W for mixing and administering medicated infusions, not primary IV therapy.

2. **What action would you take if the blood vessel you palpated for IV access had a pulse to it?**

   If the blood vessel you palpated has a "pulse" to it, it is most likely an artery. Arteries carry blood under much higher pressure than veins and pose significant bleeding hazards if punctured during IV therapy. Consequently, arteries are never used for IV therapy. In the case study, the EMT must immediately recognize that the vessel is an artery and find a new blood vessel that is a vein.

3. **What may happen if you were to start the IV and administer fluid into the patient's left arm?**

   Because the patient has had her left breast removed (mastectomy), the left arm should be avoided when establishing an IV. Removal of a breast sometimes involves the removal or resection of blood vessels and lymphatic channels that drain the arm. As a result, the administration of fluid into the arm on the same side as the mastectomy can result in edema and pain. Therefore, it is best to avoid starting an IV in this arm. If the patient has had a bilateral mastectomy (removal of both breasts), contact medical direction for further action.

CHAPTER 5

Equipment Used for Intravenous Access

RATIONALES

1. Given the presentation of the patient, where on the patient would you most likely start the IV?

   Because the patient is dehydrated and requires a large amount of IV fluid, the EMT should look for a large sturdy vein into which a larger-gauge IV catheter can be inserted. Larger veins are typically found on the forearm or in the AC region.

2. How would you know the patient has received enough IV fluid and is improving?

   When administering IV fluid for dehydration, it is critical that the EMT periodically reassesses the patient for signs of improvement. In this case, clinical signs and symptoms suggesting improvement would be a slowing heart rate, stronger radial pulse, higher blood pressure, and resolution of the confusion.

3. What would you do if you could not successfully place an 18 or larger gauge catheter into the patient?

   If a large-gauge catheter, such as a 16-gauge catheter, could not be successfully placed in the patient, the EMT should consider using a smaller-gauge catheter such as an 18- or 20-gauge. A smaller-gauge catheter is better than no IV and can be used until a larger one can be placed at a later time. Some medical authorities consider an 18-gauge IV catheter to be sufficient to administer large amounts of fluid to the patient in need.

Obtaining Intravenous Access

RATIONALES

1. Would a 14- or 16-gauge IV catheter be appropriate for this patient?

   Because the patient does not require large amounts of IV fluid, a larger-gauge IV is not necessary. Placing a larger-gauge IV catheter into a patient can be more difficult than a smaller-gauge IV, not to mention more painful. Therefore, it is important to match the appropriate-size IV catheter to the needs of the patient. In this case, a 20-gauge IV catheter is sufficient if any medication needs to be given in the future.

2. How is a TKO rate of benefit to this patient?

   Because the patient does not require large amounts of IV fluid, a TKO rate is used. TKO means to keep open, in this case, to keep the vein open. After a catheter is inserted into the vein, blood clots can form at the distal tip of the catheter. This will block the flow of IV fluid into the patient and create problems in the patient if it breaks free and lodges in the lungs (pulmonary embolism). To keep blood clots from forming, a small amount of IV fluid is continually administered through the IV at a TKO rate. A TKO rate describes delivering one drop of IV fluid every three to five seconds.

3. Why use a hand vein for the IV and not the AC, where the veins are larger and generally easier to access?

   This IV is being started because the patient has an altered mental status and does not require large volumes of IV fluid. Therefore, smaller veins found in the hand are appropriate. Although the veins in the AC are larger and may be easier to access, starting an IV in this area is not indicated and may impair the flow of IV fluid from a lower IV site if the attempt in the AC is unsuccessful. Also, any flexion of the elbow and arm may kink the IV catheter and impair the flow of IV fluid into the patient. Given the patient's presentation, it is best to start the IV lower on the extremity and leave the AC veins for situations in which large amounts of IV fluid must be rapidly administered.

Factors Affecting Flow Rate and Complications of IV Therapy

RATIONALES

1. When restarting the IV on this patient, what type of IV administration tubing would you use?

   Because the patient has been traumatically injured and may be hemorrhaging internally, you would want to select IV tubing that could administer a large amount of fluid very quickly if needed. Therefore, macrodrip administration tubing would be the IV tubing of choice. The EMT could also use blood tubing because the patient may require blood in the hospital. Even though the EMT cannot administer blood in the field, having the blood tubing already in place would eliminate the need for hospital staff to restart the IV with blood tubing, thus enabling the immediate administration of blood on arrival at the hospital. This may be a lifesaving measure in itself.

2. How do you know that the problem with the IV is infiltration and not a locally infected site?

   The hematoma, edema, and redness at the IV site, coupled with an IV that will not flow, are telltale signs that the IV has infiltrated. When an IV infiltrates, blood from the vein flows into the surrounding tissue producing the redness and hematoma. Similarly, IV fluid escapes the vein and collects in the tissue outside the blood vessel, thus producing edema. An infiltrated IV is useless and must be restarted using all new material and supplies at another site. A local infection does not produce a hematoma, although it is often accompanied by redness and some edema. Also, a local infection takes some time to become apparent and would most likely not be obvious in the time it has taken to remove the patient from the car.

3. What has happened to the vein to cause it to infiltrate?

   Infiltration occurs when the venipuncture device goes through the blood vessel wall a second time, after entering the vein originally. This creates an opening in the vein that allows the IV fluid and blood to escape from the vessel and collect in the surrounding tissues. As a result, IV fluid will not flow into the patient, making the IV site useless. Blindly "sticking" the patient with the venipuncture device or forcefully inserting the IV catheter into the vein, as well as excessive patient movement, are all causes of IV infiltration.

Calculating Volumes of Fluid and IV Flow Rates

RATIONALES

1. What would you do if you could not establish an IV with a 14- or 16-gauge IV catheter?

   If placing a 14- or 16-gauge IV catheter were unsuccessful, it would be perfectly acceptable to attempt another IV using a smaller gauge such as an 18- or even 20-gauge IV catheter. Although not optimal, an 18- or 20-gauge IV catheter would allow fluid therapy to be started, while the EMT or other advanced health care provider works on placing a larger-gauge catheter.

2. If the patient's systolic blood pressure was 92 mm Hg after the delivery of 900 milliliters of IV fluid, what action would you take?

   If the patient's blood pressure reaches 90 mm Hg systolically before all the IV fluid has been administered, the EMT would readjust the flow rate to TKO. Administering too much IV fluid may excessively increase the patient's blood pressure and dislodge naturally forming blood clots around the site of injury. Therefore, most authorities recommend administering IV fluid to the trauma patient at a set volume of 20 milliliters per kilogram or until the blood pressure is between 80 and 100 mm Hg. If all the fluid has been administered and the blood pressure is below what medical direction desires, a second IV bolus of 20 milliliters per kilogram may be ordered.

3. What would happen if the EMT used the patient's weight in pounds instead of kilograms to calculate the volume of IV fluid to be administered?

   If the EMT used the patient's weight in pounds instead of kilograms to calculate the amount of IV fluid to administer, the volume administered would be 3,600 milliliters (20 milliliters $\times$ 180 pounds) instead of 1,600 milliliters (20 milliliters $\times$ 80 kilograms). This is a tremendous increase in fluid and may be detrimental if all the fluid was administered and the patient's systolic blood increased significantly above the goal of 90 mm Hg. Therefore, it is critical that the patient's weight be converted to kilograms prior to calculating the specific amount of fluid.

Although it could be argued that as long as the EMT assessed the blood pressure and stopped the fluid bolus when the pressure reached 90 mm Hg systolically, no harm could occur. This may be true, but such technique is bad form and serves to hurt the EMT in the future should he or she be managing a patient for whom a set amount of fluid must be delivered independent of the patient's blood pressure.

Special Patient Considerations

RATIONALES

1. Given that the patient is not hypovolemic, at what rate would you administer the IV fluid and what would you specifically assess to determine whether the patient is becoming overloaded with IV fluid?

   Because the patient does not appear to be hypovolemic, a TKO flow rate is appropriate. Even though the rate is TKO, the EMT must periodically assess to determine if too much fluid is being administered and the patient is becoming overloaded. Specifically, the EMT should examine the blood pressure, breath sounds, and pulse oximetry reading. An increasing blood pressure, moist breath sounds, and declining pulse oximetry reading may indicate that too much fluid is being administered.

2. Would it be equally acceptable to not start the IV, given that the patient is no longer seizing?

   Given the patient's condition and chief complaint, it would be unacceptable to not attempt an IV on this patient, unless local medical direction does not permit it. A nonseizing patient is much easier to place an IV in than one who is seizing. Because the patient has no history of seizures but has seized, there is something dramatically wrong. IV access is an important aspect of care in the event he seizes again (as he does in the case study), and anticonvulsants must be immediately administered. Waiting for paramedics to start the IV may delay needed care and contribute to a less than desirable outcome. Follow local medical direction in such cases.

3. Why is it a good idea to keep the mother informed of what is happening, not only when starting the IV, but regarding overall care?

   When managing a pediatric patient, the EMT must always remember that the parents or caregivers are often just as distressed, if not more so, and must be included as "patients." To gain compliance with the parents or caregivers, as well as to assist the patient in remaining calm, let them know what is going on and what to expect, not only with IV therapy but with all patient care (when possible). Informed caregivers or parents are less likely to lose control and can be an asset in the delivery of emergency care to the sick or injured pediatric.

Special Procedures

RATIONALES

1. What action(s) would you take if, while changing the IV fluid bag, the exposed spike of the IV tubing fell onto the ground?

   The spike of the IV tubing is sterile and must not be contaminated. If the exposed spike contacts any surface, including the patient, it is considered contaminated and requires replacement. Failure to do so increases the patient's risk for infection because contaminates will then be introduced into the patient.

2. Why is it advantageous to use the slide clamp to stop the flow of IV fluid when changing the IV fluid bag?

   Using the slide clamp to stop the flow of IV fluid when changing the bag instead of the flow regulator (roller clamp) is advantageous because the EMT will not have to reset the flow rate.

3. Is it necessary to change the primary IV tubing any time the IV fluid bag needs to be replaced?

   When changing the IV fluid bag, it is not necessary to change the IV administration tubing. The only exception is when the spike of the IV tubing is contaminated. If this happens, the IV tubing must also be changed.

Legal Concerns and Documentation

RATIONALES

1. What is the most important piece of information related to this accusation that has been documented in the PCR?

   Although all information contained in the PCR is important, the saving grace is that the EMT documented the location where the IV was initiated. Because the IV initiated prehospital was in the left arm and not the right, this precluded the EMT from further action associated with the lawsuit. If the EMT had failed to document the location of the IV, he could have been held responsible for a complication not related to his care.

2. What may have happened if the EMT did not thoroughly document the IV therapy provided?

   If the EMT did not thoroughly document all information and care related to the IV therapy, he may have unfairly been held accountable for the complication and faced legal consequences. Therefore, it is essential that the EMT take the time to thoroughly document all information related to the IV therapy. If it is not written down, it was not done!

3. Given the information in the case study, and assuming IV therapy is within the EMT's scope of practice, could the EMT also be accused of an act of commission or omission?

   Assuming IV therapy is within the EMT's scope of practice, it does not appear that he committed an act of commission or omission. If the EMT did not start the IV when it was clearly indicated, he would have been guilty of committing an act beneath the standard of care, and therefore, an omission. If the EMT had gone above his scope of practice, for example, administering a medication, he would have committed an act of commission. If injury to the patient was the result of either of these acts, he could have been held for negligence and faced serious legal action.